VET
Downunder

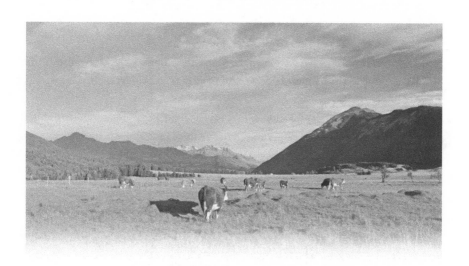

Dr Mike Small

BVSc, MACVSc

Small Animal Publishing

To my late parents, who provided the loving support,
inspiration and encouragement for me
to succeed in my rewarding career choice.
And to all our hairy four-legged friends,
large and small, who bring so much joy and
companionship to our lives.

These recollections are true.
Some veterinarians have allowed me to use their names, but elsewhere,
I have changed the names of people and their pets to protect their privacy.

Text copyright © Mike Small, 2021
Cartoons copyright © Jonathan Shih, 2021
First published 2021
ISBN 9780646831046 (pb)
ISBN: 9780646831060 (epub)

Design and layout: Cathy Larsen Design
Editing and production: Nan McNab

Contents

Introduction

Like many baby boomers, I loved James Herriot's books and the TV series All Creatures Great and Small. But unlike most, I was filled with a determination to become a veterinarian. Growing up with constant four-legged companions – family cats and dogs – and the companionship and joy they provided, I was powerfully influenced by James Herriot's humorous recollections of practice life in the Yorkshire Dales; it was to seal my future career. Being a vet has proved a rewarding and all-consuming journey, one that has certainly had its ups and downs, as any career can have, especially in the caring professions.

Benjamin Franklin once said, 'Either write something worth reading or do something worth writing.' When I read that I thought, well, I have so many good stories about what I've done, I should write them down. Many have a humorous twist, which is important in challenging times, and fun at all times. And who better to share my recollections than I myself! It's been a long time since Herriot . . .

In the beginning

I was born in Levin, Horowhenua, New Zealand, but my first eleven years were spent living in Otaki, just south of Levin, where my businessman father ran two bookshops. Everything seemed larger than life to me then. We were taught early on to make our own way and I was only nine or ten when I cycled eight kilometres from Otaki township to Otaki Beach each day after school to deliver papers.

Those years were blissfully happy with cake tins always full of my mother's weekly baking and our clothes and costumes hand-sewn. A treat was a trip to the milk bar for an ice-cream or milk-shake, or to the dairy for a white paper bag of assorted lollies we carefully selected – one cent each, or five for three cents. We spent a lot of time by or in the water, trawling for flounder off Otaki Beach, avoiding the deep end and the crab bites, or taking boat trips way out to sea.

My parents were involved in local business events and charities, which included tugs of war, sack races, egg and spoon races, and other excuses for a get-together.

We then moved back to the town of my birth for two years

when I was eleven, where my grandparents lived. My father's dad, whom we called 'Pop', used to extend his well-worn butcher's hand to welcome us, normally with a dollop of mashed potato concealed in his palm! I loved our overnight stays with my grandparents in a bed warmed by an electric blanket to partially offset the lack of insulation, and breakfast in bed the next morning.

The first hint of breakfast approaching was the sound of my grandfather scratching the burnt toast in the kitchen, followed by a whiff of the same, before my grandmother's woven cane tray with the breakfast spread arrived. After breakfast, the order of the day was a whitebaiting trip to Foxton River in the Austin A40 with whitebait nets loaded side by side on the roof rack. Lunch was always 'chargrilled' sausages cooked on a stick over an open fire, then wrapped in a piece of white bread with butter and smothered in tomato sauce. Even in those days the catch was often so small we would count the fish one by one throughout the day, but sometimes we got lucky and there were too many to count! We always ate them that night, and I can still see my nan beating up the eggs to make fritters. The whitebait were always tasty because they were so fresh.

During my childhood, our family almost always had a cat or two and a dog. Our first dog was a black cocker spaniel called Rocky. He was the archetypal high-energy cocker spaniel with his long floppy ears, waggy docked tail and mischievous disposition. We had lots of fun with Rocky, especially on family outings. The ageing cat, Tippy, wasn't so impressed with the exuberance of her canine housemate, but like many cats, begrudgingly tolerated Rocky. Tippy was the boss, as the cat often is. However, this didn't stop Rocky from constantly testing the status quo only to be put back in his place by a swipe across the nose. I've come to learn that for those planning to have both a cat and dog, it is best to raise them together as puppy and kitten. This is not always possible of course.

One morning, Rocky was missing. We found him dead in the local park. We were devastated and I still remember the moment we received the bad news. Exactly what happened to Rocky has always been a mystery; the local vet wasn't sure, without further investigation, what had killed him. As an impressionable and sensitive child, I never forgot the loss of my dog, and it was a rude awakening to the realities of owning a pet – their lifespan, already relatively short, can suddenly be cut even shorter. The heartache and grief I felt from losing Rocky no doubt helped me develop the sympathy and empathy I would need to help people through the loss of their pets, but they were hard-won qualities.

It wasn't long before we had a new puppy, Jake, a black labrador and everyone's friend. Unconditional friendliness is the rule rather than the exception for labradors – they really are great family dogs. He loved to play and follow us around, and we had many happy times over many more years than we ever spent with Rocky.

After the two years the family spent in Levin, my parents moved north to the city of Napier. I was thirteen, and stayed on with my maternal grandmother to complete term one of my first high-school year in Levin. One of my last recollections of that time was my grandmother bent double, laughing, after I was pooped on by a seagull as I prepared to bike back to school! I now remember with pleasure my grandma's glee over my small misfortune, although it was hard to appreciate at the time. Still, I took it as a sign of good luck to come. Maybe that seagull had an idea of my future profession.

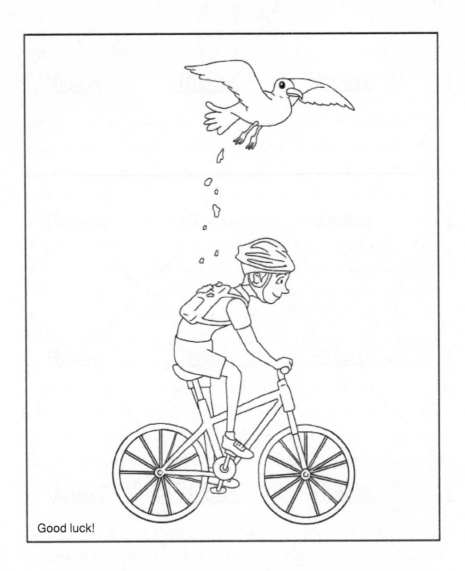

Good luck!

Napier is a beautiful, art deco city on the east coast of New Zealand's North Island. My high-school years there were the usual mix of schoolwork and the interests and distractions of teenagers. Fortunately, I had a strong aptitude for the sciences, which was handy for an aspiring veterinarian.

My sporting prowess, especially in team games, left much to be desired. Natural hand-eye coordination seemed lacking in our family, brought into stark focus by the obviously superior sporting skills of many of my classmates. I preferred more individual pursuits such as athletics, running, cycling and hiking. Pounding the hill country behind Napier city as part of the harriers club on the weekend and running eight miles over Napier's Bluff Hill on weeknights kept me fit. Wonderful tramping opportunities abounded in the scenic mountain ranges around Napier – the Kawekas, Kaimanawas and the Ruahines.

Napier's dry summers provide an ideal climate for the vineyards and orchards that dot the local landscape, but the weather can be notoriously windy. Any local cyclist can attest to this, and I have very strong memories of both a headwind cycling to school in the morning and a headwind on the way home in the afternoon. This provided very good training for the even stronger winds that managed the same 180 degree about-face during the day whilst I was at veterinary school in Palmerston North.

My family were never without a cat; in fact we often had two. Fluffy, one of our Napier cats, was exactly that. Her breed could be described as 'domestic long hair'. Regular grooming was a must to keep the knots from her coat and fortunately for us she loved the attention. This is not always the case and throughout my working life I've had to sedate or anaesthetise many cats so our nurses could groom them. The owners, after a first attempt at home, dared not risk life and limb to groom their beloved pets.

Fluffy was less biddable in another regard, and it wasn't long before she began to blossom with the telltale signs of a developing pregnancy. I was to discover many times during my career that we were not the only family whose young feline jumped the gun and got in first before their desexing appointment! When the time came, she elected to have the kittens on my parents' bed, so that proved to be educational for all the family. Five kittens! Some weeks later, after much pleading, my parents gave in and we were allowed to keep a grey one, which we named Josie. Fluffy had good genes and a nice nature so it was very easy to place the other four kittens in loving homes.

Our family dogs at the time were English and Irish setters, quite different to the happy-go-lucky labrador, but still lots of fun. These setters can be a bit skittery if not reared and handled correctly, which was good training for me. Generally it was my job to take them for a walk, or a run more like it, and as you can imagine they and I were kept fit.

It was at this time that I became infatuated with the biographies of James Herriot, a pseudonym for James Alfred Wight. For those who remember, James Herriot was an English veterinarian who practised in the Yorkshire Dales and produced no fewer than six books recounting highlights from his veterinary career. The entertaining television series All Creatures Great and Small was based on the books. Once I had read the books, front to back several times, I was determined to become a vet. I loved animals, and I had an aptitude for the sciences. My career path was sealed. It was the beginning of a lifelong passion.

I had other interests, one of which was amateur winemaking. However, despite my father kindly vacating his toolshed on no fewer than two separate occasions for winemaking, I couldn't find a ready outlet for my product. Unfortunately, despite my scientific approach, my dandelion-head, carrot, parsnip, pineapple and beetroot wine didn't have quite the receptive market I'd hoped for. Wine produced from Müller-Thurgau, Riesling-Sylvaner and Cabernet Sauvignon grapes – grape varieties grown in the 1970s – definitely produced a superior wine.

We didn't have to worry about a market for the ginger beer I brewed because that all blew up in one loud impressive explosion on a quiet summer's evening. Fortunately, the brew bottles were sealed in wooden apple boxes outside, having been banned from the house.

I set about building a rack and cloth press for pressing the juice from crushed grapes, hoping for more success. The closest I could get locally to the recommended oak to build it from was the timber of the New Zealand tanekaha or celery pine, a strong but flexible wood. With my father's help, I managed to secure grapes from a whole row of vines in the vineyard of a family friend. The quality of my homemade wine improved, and not surprisingly I found a ready outlet for my produce.

My parents owned and operated a large food business in Napier, and I and my three siblings were taught to cook from an early age. With winemaking and catering in my blood, albeit at a very amateur level, food technology seemed like a good backup plan to pursue if I wasn't accepted into veterinary science. This probably explains the slight bias towards food-related topics throughout my writing. In saying that, a lot of veterinary clinical cases do centre around the gastrointestinal system, and the inappropriate ingestion by our hairy friends of all manner of things, and the consequences that follow! Some of our most interesting clinical cases arise from the gut.

Thankfully, with hard work and determination, and some good fortune, I didn't need to implement plan B.

In training and more

In New Zealand, there is only one veterinary school, in Palmerston North. It was known as the Faculty of Veterinary Science from its first intake of students in 1963 until 1998. It then became the Institute of Veterinary, Animal and Biomedical Sciences, or IVABS.

I completed my veterinary training in the early 1980s, with a one-year break halfway through the five years of study, gainfully employed while I had a breather.

The veterinary course involved field studies in animal behaviour and I spent a fair bit of time sitting in a lambing paddock recording lambing behaviour. I undertook a literature review of feline copulation or mating – a relevant topic for a vet student! The degree course also involved farm and veterinary clinic practical components. Farm stays for a city boy were a unique experience. The hospitality of the farmers and their wives was fantastic, and I got to taste some interesting kai (Te Reo Māori word for food). I hadn't realised you could serve roast lamb and mutton in so many ways. In some cases we had it every day – hot at night and sliced cold during the day. On Sunday, though, we were treated to a beef or pork roast. I'm sure that with the advent of modern cuisine, and the range of foods available in supermarkets, the range of meals on farms is now more varied.

One farm I stayed at in the Kimbolton, Manawatu, area of the North Island was at risk of its paddocks being overrun with Scotch thistle, a common introduced weed, so I was put to work hacking and spraying them. I remember seeing the largest rhubarb plant I had ever seen planted in a sunny, well-drained, north-facing position right next to the woolshed. I asked the farmer his secret. The wry smile said it all!

It reminded me of the time when, halfway through a guided tour of the Sanitarium™ factory in Auckland, with my older sister Deidre kindly accompanying me, we were asked if we had any questions. When nobody offered any, I ventured the most intelligent question I could think of: 'So what are the Ricies made of?' I have never quite lived that one down.

I learnt some important lessons on these farm stays: learn to laugh at yourself and don't take yourself too seriously, and it's good to enjoy a laugh at someone else's expense from time to time as well.

As part of my practical farm work I spent time on a combined piggery and dairy farm. It was essential to don earmuffs before entering to feed the penned pigs. Without getting into the ethics of penned pig farming, it was certainly less than ideal. As soon as the sows saw you with the feeding barrow all hell broke loose, and it became a 120-decibel screaming match! They were gentle creatures, though, despite their voracious appetite, and they would often give you a friendly nudge. A nose peg would have been handy, but I grew accustomed to the pong and would have to deal with far worse during my career. The piggery smell was persistent, and clothes, skin and hair required a fair bit of washing and scrubbing to eliminate it. I didn't mind though. It was part of the job and I was a wide-eyed student full of hope for the future. I enjoyed my time and the farmer was a good sort with a pleasant demeanour of unflappable congeniality.

I was very lucky indeed to spend time with Harry Dewes, a well-respected horse vet in Hamilton. Harry was a delightful veterinarian who was nearing retirement. He had a keen interest in soil science and was ever ready to share his knowledge. He taught me about many of the pasture grasses, amongst other things. We would stop the car along the way and pick grasses and seed heads to be mounted in a book as part of the practical requirement. His efforts earned me brownie points with our assessing professor when we were asked to identify grasses in our vet student practical groups.

One incident stood out from this time with Harry. We visited a horse stud where Harry was to examine a young stallion for an abnormality. This required the horse to be penned and placed into a chute or crush.

The usual greetings were exchanged, along with the common banter between veterinarian and client. There was some difficulty in penning the young thoroughbred and although they had him in a loose yard, he wouldn't go into the chute so he could be examined. Various lasso ropes were tossed through the air but he either evaded them or flicked them off. I was quite intrigued by this, but the others vented their frustration with a fair bit of foul-mouthed cussing. Instant equine experts appeared from every corner of the yard to offer advice freely, but nothing seemed to be working. How could such a group of experienced horsemen have so little luck penning a young, rambunctious equine?

Finally, one of the assembled handlers, in fact the blacksmith who had been chipping in with his own suggestions, marched into the pen and up behind the horse, uttering the phrase that would pass into folklore. 'The trouble with you guys nowadays is you've got no guts!' With that the young thoroughbred lashed out and kicked the blacksmith full-force in the nether region. Bullseye!

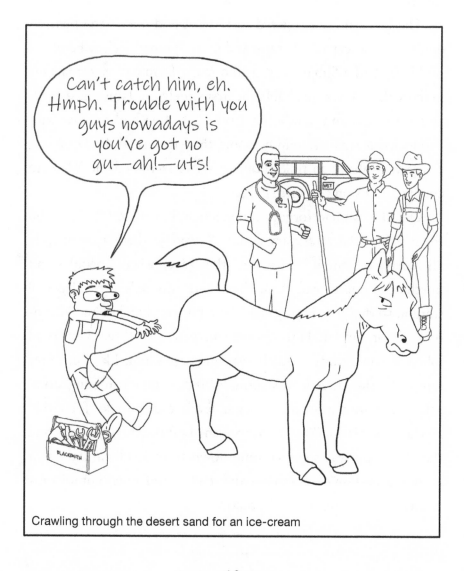

Crawling through the desert sand for an ice-cream

The now speechless victim dropped to his knees and crawled through the dirt! It must have been an agonising minute or so before he was able to draw his first breath. Even to the uninitiated it seemed that the inevitable was going to happen from the very moment he entered that pen, so there was not a lot of sympathy from the crowd, but rather a cackle of amusement, and Harry's wisecrack comment: 'Crawling through the desert sand for an ice-cream.'

The blacksmith staggered to his feet and out of the pen, no doubt to seek icepack therapy and more sympathy elsewhere!

Harry had a Subaru car, as did many farm-call veterinarians in those days. It was probably the first widely available and affordable 4WD car and handy for a vet who often had to drive into paddocks; it was less cumbersome than the usual 4WD or ute. There was plenty to talk about as we crisscrossed the Waikato country roads on our farm calls.

One day we had forgotten our lunch, having left it sitting on the bench at the veterinary clinic. Nowadays there are probably all sorts of small cafes on the way where people can purchase a bite to eat. Back then there was only a rural petrol station, so that day, Harry went in to buy our lunch. I had visions of a pie or similar. Harry soon emerged with three packets of lollies – wine gums, oddfellows, and something like pineapple lumps! By this stage it was about 2.00 pm and a rumbling stomach and plummeting blood-sugar levels didn't make for either restraint or reason. We almost polished off the three packets and the afternoon was spent coming down from a substantial sugar high! Harry didn't seem to bat an eyelid...and it was not my only culinary adventure in rural practice.

Having attended high school in Napier, I was aware of the established veterinary practices in the town before I began my hometown vet work there. 'Mixed animal' refers to a practice that services both companion animals and farm (or lifestyle) animals. Most city practices are companion animal only and many small-town or rural practices are mixed. Courtney St George was the well-known, popular and longstanding owner of one of these practices. Courtney was a Second World War veteran and had trained at Sydney Veterinary School after returning from war service. He was a real gentleman. From the beginning I had been impressed with Courtney's independence, strength of character and enthusiasm for his work. He was a master of self- discipline and determination, having adapted his skills to practise with a minimum of nursing assistance, as was common in those days. His strong work ethic impressed me, and he was a good story-teller, which I very much enjoyed. He was patient and willing to share his knowledge and experiences. We spent many hours sitting on stools in his dispensary cum tea room while he recounted veterinary, family and wartime stories.

Veterinary practice over the years has progressed at a phenomenal pace. The armoury of drugs and equipment advanced a long way during Courtney's years of practice and has progressed in leaps and bounds since. For example, in the 1980s, the main antibiotics in use were amoxicillin, tetracyclines, first-generation quinolones (just) and sulpha drugs. Now, we have potentiated penicillins and a host of others and second- and third-generation quinolones, with the unfortunate emergence of major antibiotic resistance in many cases. Courtney could remember penicillin powders and concocting his own medicines!

He had an impressive one-handed technique for anaesthetising cats and he also taught me how to single-handedly place an endotracheal tube – an anaesthetic breathing tube – into a dog or cat's windpipe. We have highly qualified veterinary nurses now who make this job much easier, but Courtney's technique is still very useful. When I look back on 'seeing practice' as it was colloquially known, there are lots of examples of how far we have come over the years.

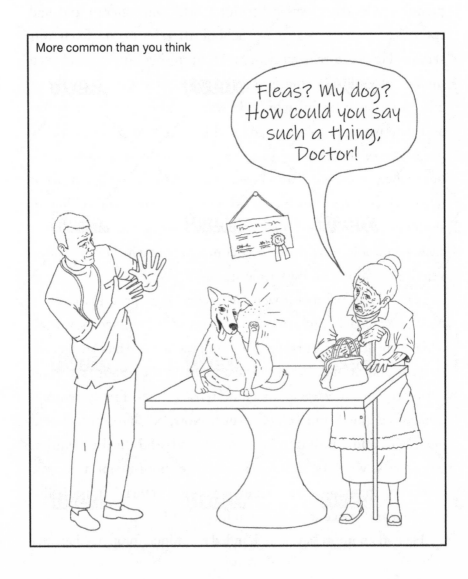

The flea treatments for cats and dogs in those days consisted of flea powders, flea sprays (just like a can of fly spray but sprayed all over the animal's coat with a fair portion of it inhaled by the person applying the spray), dips and flea collars – these products have been superseded by much more effective treatments. Now we have three- and six-month topical preparations, three-month oral tablets and no doubt in the near future injectable yearly flea treatments will become available.

Our standard skin-allergy treatment included dexamethasone and prednisone pills to suppress inflammation and the immune response. Now we have a host of therapies, including monoclonal antibody treatments, specific inflammatory pathway inhibitors, other immunotherapies, allergy-free diets and skin specialists as well! Every area of human activity and endeavour has come a long way over the years and veterinary science is no exception.

The veterinary course, like many professional courses, consists of several years of teaching to lay the foundation for the more advanced clinical years of the course. For many, those first two to three years are a challenge and involve two years of anatomy, physiology and genetics, along with other subjects.

Our genetics professor appeared to be straight out of a textbook and seemed to be on a different planet, lecturing to a group that he assumed had advanced knowledge. The Sahara had more moisture in it than those lectures!

Anatomy is an important subject for veterinary students, but two years of weekly or biweekly sessions dissecting formalin-preserved animals of various species, infused with latex, required endurance and persistence. The smell left on your clothes (despite the lab coat or overalls we wore) was a formalinised version of the pig-farm smell. Of course, despite regulations, the odd anatomy specimen would end up flying across the room, or at home in someone's bed, or planted elsewhere as a practical joke. Students will be students! However, that was rare and we were in general very respectful of our patients' former lives and the kindness of their owners in donating them to veterinary science. Our anatomy lecturers must have had degrees in patience and psychology, and in hindsight deserved a medal for their efforts. Unfortunately for them we weren't all as passionate about their subject as they were.

No pain equals no gain and our dissecting efforts were to pay dividends in the end. Nobody wants a surgeon with little or no knowledge of anatomy to operate on their animal. It always intrigued me how the specimens for our anatomy practical examinations often looked different to the specimens we dissected. Of course, no two patients have the same dimensions or appearance, and it may have had something to do with an experienced dissector preparing the specimens.

'Halfway day' marked the halfway point of the five-year veterinary degree course. The highlight of this was a celebration based around the 'vet (duck) pond', or the lake outside the veterinary building. It was the middle of winter, and some of us, myself included, ended up in the drink! On leaving the water, I noticed I was missing my prized watch and had to lodge my second insurance claim in two years, after a burglary the year before. The insurance company paid out on the legitimate claim – but refused to insure me again. Students are such bad risks! Short-sighted, I thought. I had my future ahead of me and plenty of insurance with few or any claims!

The clinical years, which were largely the fourth and fifth years, were much more rewarding in general. These were the years we had been hanging out for, during which we began to see some light at the end of the tunnel. We started to do supervised operations, such as routine desexing, and had some contact with patients and clinical cases. Any animal lover who has taken their pet to the vet and has felt woozy or light-headed in the consulting room can take heart from the knowledge that there were plenty of aspiring vets who did exactly that in the operating theatre when we started student surgery classes. Watching the colour drain from your fellow students' faces and catching them before they hit the deck should have prepared us for handling the situation when our poor unsuspecting clients 'came over all funny', but no, we were all often caught out without warning.

We also got to go out on farm calls, as the Massey University Veterinary School ran a rural practice that had a local farmer client base and generously tolerated a group of students tagging along to learn. Inevitably the calls took much longer than normal as each student often had to examine the animal and come up with some ideas about the diagnosis and treatment plan. But it was all for a good cause and hopefully the client was rewarded with good service for their patience and generosity of spirit, and maybe a discount!

As you might expect, it wasn't just academic performance that determined whether we graduated or not. Not only did we have to meet certain theoretical and practical examination requirements in each clinical subject, but attitude and readiness to practise were considerations in the decision to pass or fail a student. In the caring professions there is an expectation, and rightly so, that high standards of service and the maintenance of public confidence and trust must be upheld. Our animal patients can't speak for themselves, but we can insist they receive the same high standard of care we expect for ourselves.

Wet behind the ears

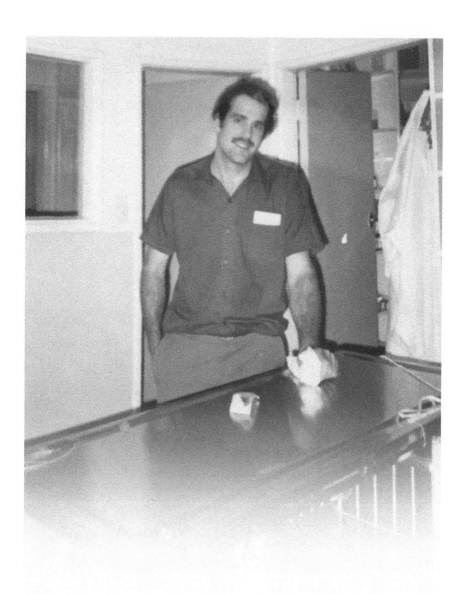

First job

Like most students in the final year of study, I felt the anxiety of whether I was going to pass my final exams, but with the right attitude to practice, and as long as my knowledge was there, I felt I should get through. I was keen to secure a job and kickstart my career. We would all scan the job-vacancy board in the vet tower, eagerly seeking that first job.

So, there it was – I blinked a couple of times and it was still there – 'Small-animal veterinarian required for veterinary practice in New Plymouth.' I applied, not expecting to get the position. I had only been to New Plymouth once in my lifetime, many years ago, and had only very vague recollections of the city. No harm in applying, I thought. I secured an interview and Richard, the jovial and studious-looking veterinarian who came to Palmerston North to interview people, must have taken a shine to me, because I got the job. Reality was about to set in. Five days after finishing at Massey, I was standing in the veterinary surgery in New Plymouth at 8.00 am on a Monday morning.

It is not necessarily an easy task for employers to take on a new graduate – they need supervision and training, which takes time and more than a modicum of patience. It's a steep learning curve for the new graduate too.

It was a good set-up and the branch practice had two-bedroom accommodation behind it. I traded in my Datsun 1200 for a newer car – a Mitsubishi Sigma sedan – for the princely sum of $23,999. With a job I was able to secure a loan – at the staggering interest rate of twenty-seven per cent! Thanks to

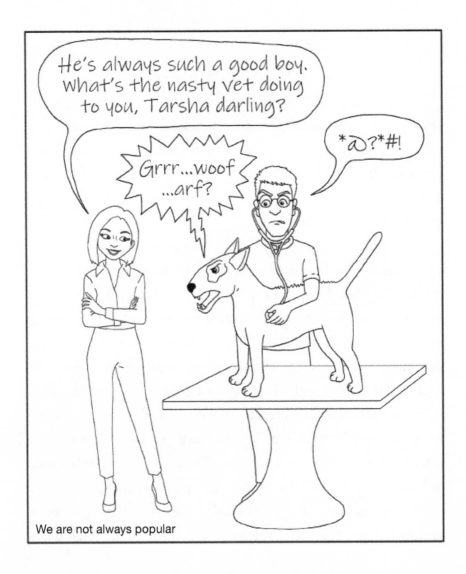

We are not always popular

the government of the day, things were pretty regulated. Someone was laughing about those rates, but it wasn't me. At least, I thought, that's the only mortgage commitment – so far.

The practice was well run by the owner's wife, Marjorie, who knew all the clients well and was a great asset to the practice. The family lived alongside the main veterinary surgery and were very welcoming. I would be happy here, but I had better be sure to meet expectations!

Richard had warned me with a grin and a chuckle that he had chihuahua breeders amongst his clients and chihuahuas were not good at whelping (giving birth naturally). What's more, they often ran into difficulty whelping in the middle of the night! I had already experienced these little 'land-sharks' and listened to industry chatter about various dog breeds. Thankfully this wasn't a fair description of the chihuahuas in Richard's practice, who were a delightfully friendly line of chihuahua, as were their breeder owners. It was a great relief because midnight calls to land-shark caesareans with worried owners would have been an induction by fire!

Light-hearted relief

Day one was induction by fire. Marjorie came through to the surgery to advise that Mrs Johnson was on her way with her three-year-old ginger, neutered male cat, Rex. Rex appeared uncomfortable, was licking 'down under' a lot and vocalising.

'That doesn't sound good, Mrs Johnson,' we heard Marjorie tell the owner. 'You'd better put Rex in his carry cage and head straight to the surgery. I'll let the vets know you're on your way.'

It wasn't long before a red-faced and flustered Mrs Johnson staggered through the surgery door with Rex. Mrs Johnson was a slight woman and Rex was the opposite. He was clearly a feline of no mean appetite, weighing in at nine kilograms. Rex's ideal weight should have been around five kilograms, suggesting that he pulled off a feeding-on-demand system at home. This isn't uncommon, but not to Rex's advantage on this occasion.

Luckily for us Rex was a friendly character, despite his distress.

What could be the problem?

Richard wasn't going to give his newbie vet any ideas, so I proceeded to examine Rex.

'His abdomen is tense and tight,' I remarked. Gentle palpation resulted in straining and distress for Rex. Not good, I thought, and straining means he could be having trouble passing a motion or urinating. 'Could this be a blocked bladder, Richard?' I asked.

A broad, acknowledging smile came over Richard's face. I'd scored my first brownie point.

Richard took Mrs Johnson aside and explained the diagnosis.

We could feel a hard, enlarged bladder inside Rex's belly, which was painful for Rex and, worse, life-threatening.

A very worried expression came over Mrs Johnson's face.

'Oh dear, Mr Drummond. I knew something bad was up and I'm pleased I was home to see this as I was heading out to my handicraft group this morning. I know he's in good hands, Mr Drummond. You'll see him right ... won't you.'

Richard assured Mrs Johnson that this condition could generally be successfully treated, but it was an emergency, and Rex needed attending to straight away. His kidney function might be affected as well, but that would generally normalise with fluid therapy and treatment. Rex needed an anaesthetic so we could unblock his urethra and bladder.

'Unblocking' involved giving Rex an anaesthetic and attempting to gently insert a lubricated, fine catheter into his penis to flush the plug that was blocking the urethra back into his bladder so he could urinate again. It was not without risk. Rex would need to stay with us for a few days until he could urinate on his own again.

'But why has this happened, Mr Drummond? He only has the best food – the most expensive cuts of red meat and biscuits.'

'Well, Mrs Johnson, despite the diet, there are a few reasons we think this happens. To help prevent a future blockage, Rex will need a special prescription diet. His weight wouldn't be

27

helping either as extra fat is probably narrowing his urethra and cats' urethras are narrow at the best of times. I'll bet he doesn't drink much either.'

'Funny that, Mr Drummond. He doesn't.'

'Well, Mrs Johnson, with few exceptions cats in general aren't big drinkers, which doesn't help. The more they drink, the more dilute the urine, which means it's less likely that debris will accumulate into a plug that blocks the urethra. We'll also need to make Rex's urine more acidic and with a lower magnesium content and we achieve that by feeding prescription food. I suspect Rex will have no problem eating his new diet!'

'No, I don't think that will be a concern, Mr Drummond. He has no trouble with his appetite.'

So, we moved Rex through to the surgery and started him on an intravenous drip and collected bloods. Fortunately, the blood test told us his kidney function and electrolytes were reasonably normal. This was a helpful start. We gave Rex light sedation and some pain relief before his anaesthetic.

'OK, Mike, it's up to you now,' Richard said.

I hadn't unblocked a bladder before, but this was the time to get started!

'Off you go, Mike, and I'll be right here to help as required.'

Off I went.

There are some challenging conditions that new veterinarians must learn to treat. Extruding the limp end of a cat's penis while he's under anaesthetic and passing a fine catheter into the small blocked 'bullseye target tip' is definitely one of them. With the helpful but slippery lubricant applied, the elusive customer stubbornly slid backwards into its sheath ... a slippery-pole type scenario.

Richard was ready with a syringe of saline to flush the plug of debris once I got the catheter end firmly inside the penile tip. This proved challenging to say the least.

Richard was impatiently waving the syringe about and occasionally squirting saline for effect, which only added to my frustration.

Perhaps if I moved closer I could see better . . . so I stooped lower, closer to my target. Good, this seemed to be working at last, and Richard managed to squirt a little saline from the syringe up the catheter that was now thankfully sitting in the penile urethra.

Richard told me to put a little pressure on the bladder through the abdominal wall to check if any urine was flowing from the end of the penis.

There was a sudden WHOOSH and a warm stream of blood-tinged urine shot out, spraying the nearest solid object – my face!

Richard burst into fits of laughter, which seemed to go on for a considerable amount of time. I realised that maybe I'd been set up, but I didn't mind as we'd achieved a successful outcome for Rex. The urine was soon wiped away and I wasn't the only one relieved that my first veterinary intervention had been successful.

Rex was much more comfortable, and went home a few days later. As expected, he had no problem eating his prescription food. Mrs Johnson was a very happy woman and so pleased to have her boy back home and recovering. Luckily for us she was also a good cook and we were rewarded for our efforts with a tasty homemade banana cake.

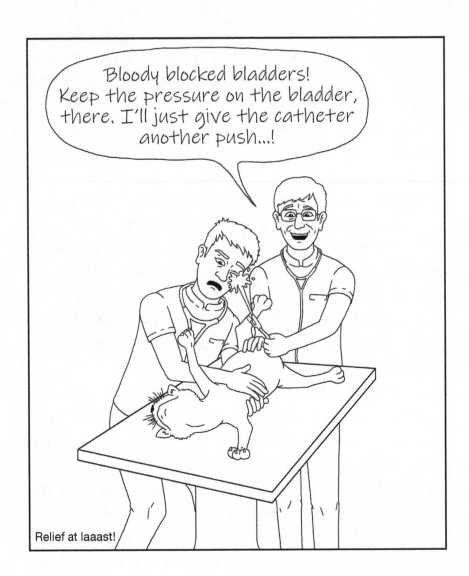

Relief at laaast!

Live and learn

It proved to be an interesting time in the branch practice. In the mornings, I would transport any surgical patients to the main surgery for their procedures. After the morning's surgery, in the early afternoon, we returned to the branch practice where I would practise solo for the afternoon.

I was the receptionist and veterinary nurse, answering calls and giving advice, as well as being the veterinarian and salesperson for small-animal products. The practice was not busy nor profitable enough to sustain a veterinary nurse, a situation that has by and large changed nowadays where most clinics employ qualified veterinary nurses. It was difficult to offer a full service practising solo.

The phone went and I answered it.

'Good afternoon. Is that the vet?'

'Yes, it is. Mike Small here. How can I help you?'

'Oh, thank goodness, it's Mrs Titter here. I'm ringing about my cat, Rastus. He hasn't eaten today and has a lump on his back near the base of his tail. He seems very unhappy and he won't let me near him to have a look. I did hear a fight the other day and

31

Rastus was outside. He's a bit of a fighter, Mr Small. I think I need to bring him to see you.'

'Yes, I agree he needs to be seen, Mrs Titter. Bring him down now if that suits.'

'That sounds fine, Mr Small. I'll be on my way.'

It wasn't long before a well-dressed and slightly flustered older woman appeared at the door with a cardboard cat carry box in one hand and a purse in the other. I opened the door and ushered them in.

Rastus was not too pleased about being confined in his carry box. He was vocalising constantly with plaintive meows and trying to paw his way out of the box. Ginger paws repeatedly appeared through the slit at the bottom ends of the box. This looked quite comical, but wouldn't be too good if it were followed by a cat shooting out the bottom.

I hastened Mrs Titter and Rastus through to the examination room before more than a paw appeared. Mrs Titter was visibly relieved as she placed the weighty box on the consulting room floor.

As I opened the leaves of the cat box, Rastus's head shot out. Judging from the historic wounds and scars on his head there was no doubt he was a seasoned fighter. The deteriorating appearance over time of many a warrior cat's head and ears is evidence of their territorial spats, and Rastus was no exception! Or, as the clients often put it . . . this cat's cost me a 'bloody fortune'. Forked and often misshapen ears, sometimes with small flaps of previously shredded and healed skin, are common.

However, Mrs Titter was not concerned about cosmetic or financial matters and was more focused today on poor Rastus's welfare.

Although a friendly cat, he was very anxious about this unusual encounter.

'Now, let's have a look at him,' I said. I lifted Rastus onto the examination table.

It didn't take long to see what Mrs Titter was talking about. Rastus had a swelling over the area of his right rear rump just in front of his tail-base. It felt very fluidy and the skin was definitely warmer than usual. A matted clump of fur provided the telltale clue – a cat fight infection or abscess.

Cats' mouths and teeth have their share of undesirable bacteria and a cat bite injects them under the skin where they can quickly form an infection. Cats' skin is also very loosely attached to the underlying connective tissues, which means abscesses can spread quite quickly and become very large over a relatively short period of time, especially if unnoticed and not promptly treated. Under furry or fluffy coats, bite wounds and abscesses can prove a challenge to detect early in many cases.

I mentioned to Mrs Titter that I would give Rastus pain relief and an antibiotic injection and that he would need to stay at the clinic to have his abscess treated. 'If you wouldn't mind, Mrs Titter, just hold onto Rastus for a minute while I draw up the injections,' I said.

Mrs Titter had gone a little quiet but acknowledged my request as I turned to the cabinet on the wall to draw up the required drugs into syringes.

It was a fine day outside I noted, glancing out the side window, although a little stuffy in the examination room. Air-conditioning was not common in those days, unlike now where most premises are air-conditioned, and for very good reason.

'All OK, Mrs Titter?' I asked, as I drew up the solutions.

As I started to turn around I heard a resounding thump.

I spun around quickly to discover Mrs Titter's limp form lying prostrate on the floor of the examination room and the rear end of Rastus disappearing out the small side window, which unfortunately was ajar.

The scene unfolding before me was not a pretty one!

My immediate concern was for Mrs Titter who was out cold on the floor. I managed to prop her up and luckily she came around quickly; apart from the expected pallid appearance, she

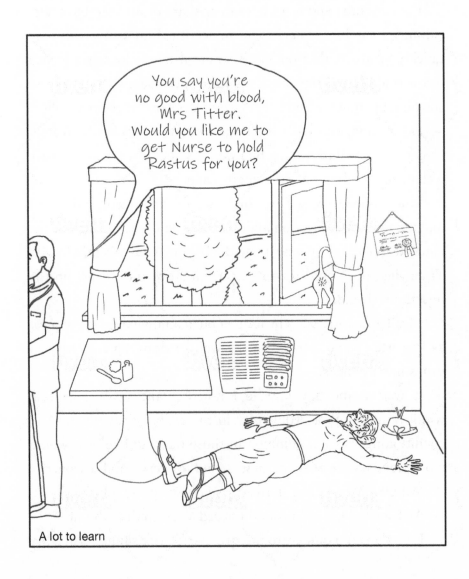

A lot to learn

seemed uninjured. Thank goodness for that, I thought. I sat her up and offered her a glass of water and the colour gradually returned to her face.

Now I could turn my attention to the escapee. Best to track him by the same route he had taken, although I was not going out the window! He had gone out the window, over a high wall and into the back alley behind the adjacent dairy.

I headed out and climbed over the wall into the alley. There he was holed up in the back corner. That was lucky, I thought, although he was none too pleased to see me and let out a hiss and growl as I approached. I thought for a minute I should retreat to the surgery for reinforcements, but he would be unlikely to be there on my return, making matters worse.

I managed to corner Rastus and blindly (or foolishly) lunged towards him and grabbed him. The wise amongst you may foresee what happened next.

Rastus, in his hyped-up, adrenaline-fuelled fight or flight response (unfortunately for me in the reverse order that day) opted to exact his pent-up revenge. He had had his flight out the window, over the high wall and into the alleyway. Now it was time for the fight, and I was the unfortunate opponent.

Rastus let fly with all the teeth and claws in his armoury on my clutching hands. Blood spewed forth, along with a few cuss words and cries of agony, before I managed to get a good grip on him. I beat a hasty retreat through the dairy and back to the surgery, much to the consternation and concern of several dairy patrons. I finally secured Rastus in a surgery cage and gave him his antibiotic and pain relief.

Mrs Titter was sitting quietly in the waiting room. I managed to wash and bathe my wounds, which luckily didn't require suturing and didn't become infected in the days that followed. Finally some calmness and control was restored.

I had learnt very quickly and the hard way the essentials of Client Relations and Animal Handling 101:

1. Keep a close eye on the demeanour of your client while in the consulting room and be aware of white-coat syndrome.
2. Keep a close eye on the demeanour of your patient while in the consulting room and be aware of white-coat syndrome.
3. Do not leave windows, doors (and cupboards, etc.) open or ajar, however small the opening, in your veterinary premises.

Rastus made a good recovery.

Dinner time

It wasn't long before news got around that there was a new vet at the branch practice.

One fine summer afternoon the bell rang. I went into the reception area to be met by a smart young woman. We exchanged pleasantries and I asked how I could help, to which she politely announced, 'Thank you, but I haven't come in for veterinary advice today.'

This was a little unusual and I wondered if she needed some assistance with a vehicle breakdown or directions. I didn't have to enquire further as she soon explained the reason for her visit.

'No, no, I heard there was a new vet in town, and I've come to ask you out to dinner!'

Well, that was unexpected, but of course a welcome surprise. I hadn't been in town long and was learning the ropes of a new job that was becoming all-absorbing. I didn't really know anyone apart from my workmates in town.

Although I hadn't had time to collect my thoughts at this point I couldn't see any harm in accepting this kind offer. And so, with date and time in hand for our dinner appointment, and address noted, I watched as she disappeared out the door.

The dinner appointment went very well, and although Rachel didn't have any animals herself for me to treat, it was nice to have some respite from the business of learning a new job, settling into a new career, and to spend some pleasant leisure time with a new companion I happened to meet at work!

New Plymouth was working out well for me as a newbie. I was finally out in the real world and settling in just fine.

Midnight solo

The branch clinic was in a small set of retail shops on a busy sub-
urban road, so it was handy enough to locate and conveniently
placed.

Luckily my dwelling was out the back away from the road, so
I could get some kip in between fielding after-hours calls in the
middle of the night.

The phone rang in the early hours of a weekday morning. It
was Marjorie.

'Mike ... I've just had a call from Miss Beamish. One of her
chihuahua bitches has started whelping and is having trouble in
second-stage labour – she's been straining for half an hour with
no result. Can you get dressed and come on down to the main
clinic?'

With a feeling of dread, I quickly got dressed and headed
down the road for fifteen minutes to what was to be the first of
many middle-of-the-night call-outs over the years. (It was always
2.00–3.00 am.)

I was more excited than fearful as I knew Richard would be
there to assist. Richard was already in the surgery getting out the

gloves, lube, and a small pair of whelping forceps. He seemed as relaxed and jovial as usual and I could only imagine that these call-outs had become routine for him regardless of the hour.

It's amazing how often emergencies wait until the middle of the night to present themselves . . . call it Sod's Law. I'll bet pet owners think the same. It's better to have youth on your side for these calls as you often have a full day of surgery the next day. Fortunately for most of us now we have dedicated after-hours clinics, meaning a fresh vet to attend these middle-of-the-night calls, rather than a sleepy-eyed animal doctor raised from the depths of slumber! Nonetheless, we always rise to the occasion as it is usually something worthy of the call.

Marjorie had an uncanny ability to sort the genuinely urgent call from that which can wait until morning, so I knew if the phone rang it needed attention. Nowadays, I wouldn't be able to sleep well knowing the phone might sing its not-so-merry tune in the middle of the night.

Miss Beamish was well used to this situation by now and knew that the sterile kit would already be laid out for the emergency caesarean, if a forceps-assisted delivery was not possible.

Our patient was looking a little exhausted and apprehensive, with good reason.

Her mum was relaxed, considering the situation. Richard performed an examination and asked for my assessment. With a gloved and lubricated finger I performed a vaginal examination. By the time second-stage labour is underway there needs to be a reasonable width of pelvic canal (some relaxation and enlargement of this occurs close to birth) to allow natural birth to occur.

I thought the pelvic canal felt narrow so I cautiously said, 'There doesn't seem much room there for a pup to pass, Richard.'

Richard's knowing nod conveyed his thinking . . . suspicions confirmed.

But we still needed to know how many pups there were. The fewer the pups the larger they're likely to be, which complicates any disparity between pup size and pelvic width or birth canal even more. Poor Jasmine. We took an X-ray and to add weight to our suspicions there was only one pup present. There was no way Jasmine was going to give birth naturally to that whopper.

We had no choice but to perform an emergency caesarean.

'I'm sorry, Joyce. There's only one pup and it's a biggy. It'll have to be a caesarean I'm afraid.'

Joyce gave a knowing and resigned nod and exclaimed, 'I thought as much. Well, you'd better get on with it then.'

So we connected Jasmine to an intravenous drip and gave her some calcium and light sedation.

Speed is of the essence between administering the anaesthetic and removing the pup, so we worked quickly. The bigger the dose of anaesthetic and the longer the time between induction (first giving the anaesthetic) and removing the pup – the less likely the pup is to survive. Fortunately, even though I was a newbie, I'd developed reasonable surgical skill in my training and I managed to remove the pup promptly from Jasmine and bring it into the outside world. Lots of careful towelling, clearing of the airway, oxygen and warmth usually manage to resuscitate all but the most distressed or over-term pup. Luckily we now have even better anaesthetics than in the 1980s and this helps pup survival. As is no doubt the case in the human field, there is still a fair bit of debate around drug use in the pre, peri and postnatal periods and this will probably continue until we have drugs that have an exceptional safety profile in all settings.

Joyce was pleased to have a healthy live pup, but of course she would have preferred a few more puppies to help pay the after-hours vet bill, rather than a solo 'gold-plated' fellow. More often than not these single pups were named after expensive labels or precious metals and given that they had the whole milk bar to themselves and no competition, not only were they of high birth weight, they were also remarkably 'good doers'.

I thought that Richard was very reasonable with his fees. This was often the case in those days, and of course it often applies now, where it's a balance between what the loyal client can afford, or stomach to pay, and the goodwill of the 'I'm not in this for the money' veterinarian. And that is often the philosophy of veterinary and no doubt medical services – we are there to help our patients, not primarily to make money. Pet insurance does help nowadays.

The satisfaction is in the successful outcome and happy patient and client, not in the remuneration. The remuneration follows if you do your job well.

Flambé

Richard had a good sense of humour. He obviously enjoyed a laugh at someone else's expense, as most of us do, but he could also laugh at himself and never took himself too seriously. This is a good way of dissipating stress of course as there are certainly plenty of tense moments and situations in the caring professions.

Richard often undertook a supervisory role at the surgery. He would do the consulting but was keen to let his young vets do the surgery and was always on hand to assist and provide guidance. This suited me fine. I was keen to develop my skills, being a new graduate, and what better way to do it but under the guidance of a skilled and experienced vet.

In the 1980s smoking indoors was neither banned nor frowned upon. Richard was a smoker and very commonly had a roll-your-own or ready-made on the go in the surgery. Those of us who grew up a few years ago were pretty used to a lit cigarette placed on the edge of a consulting table while the examination was undertaken, to be returned to once the examination was finished. Wisps of cigarette smoke permeating the air were not uncommon.

This day was no exception. It was one of my first knee surgeries and I was keen to get some expert guidance to help me through a procedure I had seen many times. I'd spent the evening before swotting up on it. We had anaesthetised our patient and clipped the affected limb and the nurse had prepped the leg for surgery. This involved shaving the hair from the limb, and cleaning as necessary, then in those days methylated spirits was applied followed by a tincture of iodine solution. This served to remove any dirt, debris and sebum and substantially reduce the bacterial count on the skin and helped to prevent infection. Preparation of the skin is similar nowadays although generally with more effective skin preparations.

I started the procedure and all was going well. I called on Richard for advice as he was leaning against the sink in the corner drawing on a roll-your-own cigarette. I glanced over and he was having a couple of last sucks on the cigarette before coming to assist. He nonchalantly tossed the smouldering butt into the sink. A whoosh of bluey-purple flames erupted behind him and he gave a loud cry. A very startled and slightly singed Richard eventually made his way over to assist me. He was quick to see the humour in the situation, and once we had regained some composure, I returned to the important task at hand. It seems the bottle of methylated spirits had been spilt in the sink and not rinsed out. This would not be my last flaming encounter in a veterinary surgery.

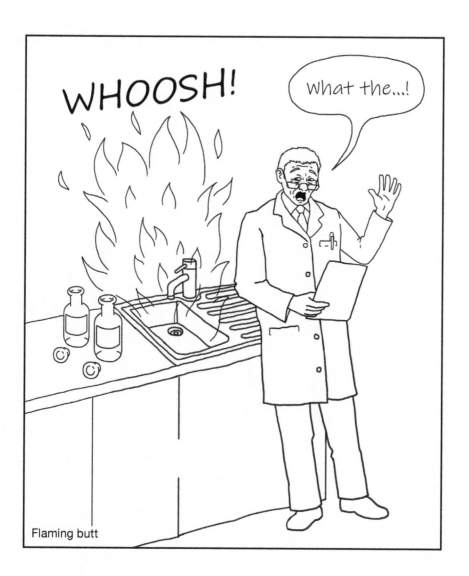

Flaming butt

Mixed practice

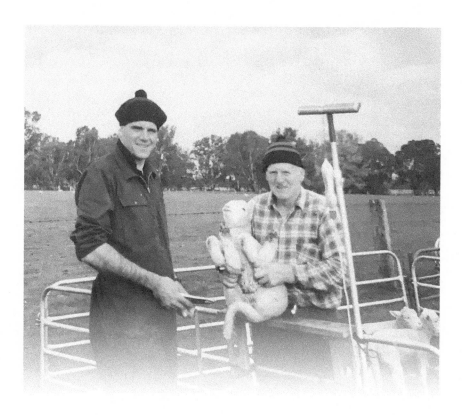

Creatures great and small

I had only been in New Plymouth for five months when my father rang and said that an opportunity to work in my home city of Napier had come up. The veterinarian I had 'seen practice with', Courtney St George, was looking to retire in the near future. Well, this was a little sooner than I had imagined but it was an opportunity to consider seriously. On the one hand I still had a lot to learn and I did not want to leave my first job after such a short period, especially as I was enjoying it and Richard and Marjorie were good to me and pleasant to work for. It did not take me long to decide, however.

Fortunately, they understood, and it was not long (one month) before I was heading to Napier to start life in a mixed-animal practice. Now 'mixed' means the practice services small and large animal clients ... companion animals, lifestyle and farm animals.

Of course, this was to be a challenge. Being a townie and reasonably fresh out of vet school I had some reservations about servicing many farmer clients who had a longstanding relationship with a veterinarian of many years' experience. However, I knew that I could rise to the challenge and fortunately Courtney was to stay on for a year or two before I took over. The enthusiasm and energy of youth, a good work ethic and the motivation of running your own business certainly helped me.

Napier sits in the agricultural fruit-bowl of northern Hawke's Bay. It has a pleasant coastal climate and is situated on the eastern aspect of the central North Island. Vineyards, horticulture, and farming predominate locally and with a population around 65 000 it is easy to get around the friendly local community.

I felt at home in Napier with a good support network, family ties, and friends and acquaintances from my high-school years. The veterinary practice had a good reputation and there was still, despite Courtney nearing retirement and local competition, about 150 farmer clients on the books. I headed up there in my newly purchased car with my puppy Wesley, a black and white pedigree fox terrier. Wesley was full of energy and loved to nose soccer balls around the backyard and chase cats if given the chance, as many terriers do. I'd better watch that tendency I decided – not very acceptable for a veterinarian's dog in particular!

I was to stay nearly ten years in Napier and I have many very fond memories, great experiences, and stories to recount.

Virus virulence

At veterinary school we had a pathology professor named Bob Jolly, who was an extremely knowledgeable, dedicated teacher and researcher. He has done a lot of ground-breaking research on various animal diseases, which has had an immense effect on the performance of animal industries and on the understanding of the diseases in humans. Over the years he has received many awards for his work, including the New Zealand Order of Merit in 2005.

As a teacher, Prof Jolly had a certain teaching style that favoured those who were fully attentive rather than those who were, shall we say, disruptive in class. However, Prof Jolly was a very fair man and if you approached his subject with anything near the passion for, and knowledge of, pathology he had, then you had nothing to fear. My final practical exam in pathology was reasonably short because he could see that I had good knowledge of his subject. I enjoyed the topic, and it was easy to understand Prof Jolly's pathology, because it was delivered with such enthusiasm and dedication. Besides, the consequences of not comprehending might be somewhat uncomfortable!

Poor old Bob's office was the recipient of a coating of whipped cream and hundreds and thousands at the end of the veterinary degree final year by two students he knew well. I'm not sure of the consequences for them, but he appeared to take it in good humour.

Of course, many of our lecturers were outstanding but none stood out as quite such a character as Prof Jolly.

Prof Jolly's lectures on canine distemper virus and canine parvovirus were delivered with the warning: 'You will see these diseases, particularly distemper, in your working career. We have had outbreaks of canine distemper virus and it will happen again.'

Canine distemper is prevented by vaccination, but it has some similarity to the rabies virus unfortunately. Many patients who get it die, and it has a mortality rate around fifty per cent, and even higher in young dogs. Affected patients often present with variable symptoms of fever, conjunctivitis, nasal discharges, involuntary twitching or gastrointestinal signs, and the disease often progresses to pneumonia or seizures or both. It is not a pleasant disease. Fortunately, it does not infect humans.

Unfortunately, when I arrived, Napier was in the middle of an outbreak of dog distemper virus.

Prof Jolly's words resounded in my ears . . . and it had not taken long unfortunately. I certainly got to see this nasty disease firsthand. We had queues of clients with their dogs lined up outside the clinic door for vaccination.

Sadly, because the disease had not been seen for a while, many clients had not had their dogs vaccinated, or their vaccinations were overdue. Worse, the practice bordered on an area where a lot of dogs had not been vaccinated at all, so we saw more than our share of clinical distemper virus cases. Although the virus does not survive long outside the patient, there are many asymptomatic carriers, therefore vaccination is essential and is now widespread in the Western world.

The good news is, we had quite a few successful recoveries, after ten to fourteen days of antibiotic treatment for the secondary bacterial infections.

Fortunately, I have not personally seen or treated a case of distemper virus infection since then and long may it continue.

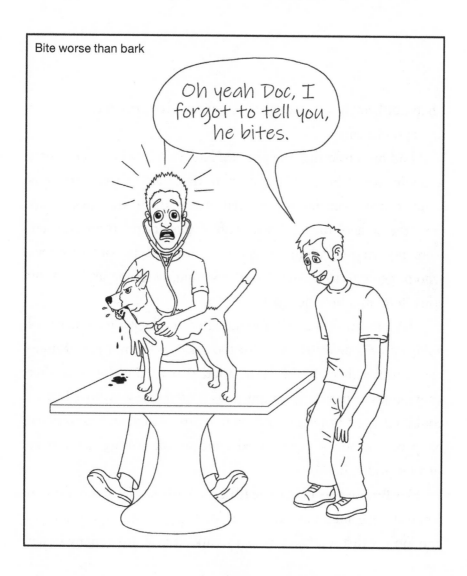

Heart in the right place

I had not been at the practice long when Mrs Brown came in for an appointment.

I had been told that the practice had a client who rescued cats and who was a bit of a character. In those days there weren't as many rescue agencies nor regulations as there are now. Apart from the Society for the Prevention of Cruelty to Animals, there were not many voluntary good-Samaritan-type organisations who in general do a great job of rescuing, desexing and treating stray, feral and homeless pets.

Mrs Brown was a self-appointed cat rescuer with a heart of gold; she was definitely in it for the cats. As the mother of nineteen children herself she understood rearing and looking after young ones! Financially strapped, as is often the way, Mrs Brown could not raise funds on-line from generous benefactors as often happens nowadays. Social media means the fishing net can be cast far and wide.

Mrs Brown was in her late fifties or early sixties, with a somewhat dishevelled appearance, her long grey wispy hair untamed and loosely thrown back from a wrinkled face. Like many of her generation, she appeared to have had all her teeth removed to save on dental expenses, however, finances or will had not extended to prosthetic enhancement regrettably. Her clothing was often a colourful afterthought that appeared to have been thrown onto her robust, generously proportioned if somewhat sagging frame. Her unique tomcat fragrance often filled the room indicating her presence before she came into view. Mr Brown occasionally accompanied his wife on her visits and was a waif of a man with white hair and whiskers who always appeared to be wearing his trademark pom-pom topped, hand-knitted woollen hat. A favourite was the rainbow knit that perfectly matched the rainbow-knitted jersey he was often wearing. The Browns' vehicles were as colourful as their owners, and could often be heard approaching because of a telltale hole in the muffler or a screeching fan belt cacophony.

Today's vehicle was the trusty Ford Prefect 100 or 107E. If it had not been for a complete lack of sport performance, this model could have passed for a local stock car. Battered and dented multi-coloured body panels indicated that the inside of the car was not likely to be any more presentable, but it functioned as a necessary workhorse until it could go no more and had to be replaced.

Mrs Brown was a happy soul and content with her lot in life. Often, one of the clan would appear in tow, carrying one or more cages of unwell cats.

Rescue cats have normally had a bad beginning and are often clinically affected by and carriers of cat flu. Their poor state of nutrition and immunity, as well as early exposure to cat flu when kittens, can set them up for a lifetime of problems. Some respond well to treatment, but others never fully recover and require ongoing treatment, if they respond at all.

Mrs Brown's cats were no exception.

On this particular day, there she was, sitting in the waiting room on the edge of the seat with a sneezing mother cat called Girl who was having difficulty breathing. We hastily ushered Mrs Brown and Girl into a consulting room to limit any spread of the virus to other patients.

'Afternoon, Mrs Brown, how are you today?'

'Not bad Mr Small,' Mrs Brown replied in her slightly lisping toothless drawl. 'I say, Girl here's not too good, she's come over all funny today. She wasn't too bad yesterday, but she hasn't touched her mince this mornin' and when she ain't eatin' I know things are bad. Snuffly 'n' all too. Can't breathe too good neither. Wotta' ya reckon?'

'Yes, I can see she's unwell, Mrs Brown. Has she been breathless like that for a while?' I replied, noting that the cat had quite laboured breathing with marked abdominal effort.

'Nup, just got real bad today. Mind, she wasn't too flash last night neither.'

I listened to her lung sounds which were raspy and laboured. Her temperature was elevated as well, and she had a bit of a cough. She certainly was sneezing and had serous conjunctivitis. Her fluid balance was not too good either and she was becoming dehydrated.

Girl had the snuffles, or feline viral rhinotracheitis, but it appeared to have moved to her lungs now and she was fighting off pneumonia, if it was not already present.

Although Mrs Brown's finances were limited, I suggested we keep Girl in isolation at the hospital, place her on an intravenous drip, administer antibiotics, anti-inflammatories, multivitamins, antiviral and supportive therapy. Besides, Girl was a lovely cat and despite her illness, was purring and rubbing herself against us as we examined her. She had lost her appetite so it would be a good idea to hand- or syringe-feed her. These cases often benefited from steam inhalation to ease nasal congestion. Although antibiotics are not commonly administered for flu in humans, or for the common cold, they are normally necessary with cat snuffles because it is the secondary bacterial infections that can result in lifelong complications or death.

It was several days before Mrs Brown was able to come and take her cat home. She arrived with the usual fanfare to collect Girl, who had certainly recovered enough to go home on medications with good home care.

Of course, Girl was not the only cat under Mrs Brown's care and the numbers grew to well over twenty before, unfortunately, steps had to be taken to reduce this number for welfare reasons.

Her heart was in the right place. Every practice has one or two Mrs Browns in some form or other. Fortunately, now, many organised charities and welfare agencies can often accommodate and treat stray or rescue cats. The big-hearted kitty Samaritans like Mrs Brown, who often have very limited finances and inadequate housing for these high-needs cats, can take a break.

I cannot leave Mrs Brown without recounting one last colourful incident.

I had employed for a period of six to twelve months, a very educated upper-middle-class English locum, with a wicked sense of humour. On his first day of work, John was initiated into the practice by a visit from Mrs Brown. She was particularly flustered that morning and had obviously rushed out of the house after dressing quickly and was looking very dishevelled. After the usual consultation for the semi-emergency, and as she was leaving the consulting room, Mrs Brown accidentally dropped her car keys on the floor near the door. It was a big consulting room and John was standing to the side of the consulting table on the other side of the room watching Mrs Brown leave. As Mrs Brown reached forward, bending her body from the hips, her skirt shot high into the air to reveal the full extent of her panty-less or commando-style unbridled womanhood! It would be fair to say John's jaw dropped; he had certainly seen more than his fair share of Mrs Brown.

Courtney

I was very lucky to have such an experienced vet to learn from during the eighteen months before Courtney's retirement. I was able to master all sorts of large-animal procedures, which I had previously only seen written about in lecture notes: pregnancy-testing cattle, gelding horses and vasectomising rams to be used as 'teasers' to indicate which ewes were ready to mate, to name a few. It was a steep learning curve. Most of Courtney's teachings were peppered with practical tips and humorous anecdotes from years of rural practice. Courtney's dry sense of humour and wit made the experience even more colourful.

I was intrigued with Courtney's single-handed technique for anaesthetising cats. Normally a nurse holds the cat and raises the vein on one of the front legs for the vet to then inject the anaesthetic into it. Courtney, however, would face the cat, hold the right foreleg with his left hand just below the elbow, raise the cephalic vein by placing pressure on it with his thumb, then inject the anaesthetic agent into it using his right hand. After the anaesthetic was slowly injected, the cat (or dog) could then be intubated (have a breathing tube inserted) using a single-handed technique again before the tube was connected to the anaesthetic machine. Naturally, the success of this 'solo' technique depended entirely on a sedated and co-operative patient, but it wasn't often he had to call for assistance. If the patient was inclined to nip, it was better for the safety of all concerned to abort this technique early, before the first-aid cabinet was required. Nowadays it is routine to have the assistance of many more well-trained veterinary nurses and there is little need for this handy technique.

When Courtney eventually retired, I decided to employ a new veterinarian. This proved to be difficult, as even in those days and more so now, veterinarians were in short supply. Eventually I managed to secure a new graduate who was happy to move back to his hometown of Napier. Employing someone with limited practical experience was always a little more difficult than employing an experienced vet, but I had just been there myself and knew that a young vet could learn quickly.

A pound and a half of chihuahua

Rosie was a delightful chihuahua, and I have met many over the years.

Joyce was a kind-hearted, portly, middle-aged woman who had a soft spot for animals and provided a loving home for those who were unwanted. She was not on Mrs Brown's scale, but there were often two or three canine companions sharing Joyce's home, and they were always smothered with affection.

I was forewarned over the phone. 'Mr Small, a friend of mine has asked me to take on a little dog who may need some veterinary attention. She is such a lovely wee girl, can you help me?'

'Of course, Joyce,' I replied, 'that's what I'm here for – I'm only too happy to assist.'

'Oh great, I'll see you tomorrow, then, when I bring Rosie in for a check-up. I'm off to pick her up shortly.'

I wondered briefly what veterinary attention this latest addition to her family needed, but was happy to wait until tomorrow to find out.

Joyce duly arrived and I escorted her into the consulting room, but I could not see any Rosie with her.

'Hello, Joyce, how are you? You haven't brought Rosie with you today then?'

With that, Joyce opened her overcoat and out of the inside pocket a tiny head appeared. It was Rosie.

'Ah, I see. Goodness, there's not much of her is there.'

In fact, we popped Rosie on the scales and she only registered seven hundred grams. Just over a pound and a half of butter!

Rosie was a very friendly girl, but a little apprehensive with mild shakes, which is not unusual for animals visiting the vet clinic. She settled a little with some patting and soothing words. Rosie appeared to have a slightly swollen stomach or abdomen, and this was the problem Joyce had come for today.

'Her boobies and her privates are swollen too, Mr Small,' Joyce announced.

'Oh yes, I can see that, Joyce,' I replied.

Rosie was eight years old and it turned out she was one of four puppies and had been the runt of the litter. It was not uncommon to have a notably smaller dog in a litter of puppies. It is thought that a runt is the result of poor placentation or a poor implantation of the placenta in the uterus. This results in a pup with a lower birth weight. Some runts can have more health problems, but not necessarily. They need to be watched closely as it can be difficult for them to compete with stronger pups for the milk bar and the mother's attention.

Rosie had evidently had a few health problems as a newborn and very nearly died, but with lots of care and attention she pulled through.

I examined Rosie and I could feel an internal lump towards the back of her abdomen.

I discussed my findings with Joyce and suggested we run blood tests and take X-rays to investigate this further. Joyce agreed.

Fortunately, Rosie's tests came back OK, and I decided the most likely diagnosis might be a growth on her ovaries or uterus which was producing hormones that resulted in the swollen privates.

I phoned Joyce and advised it was best to have Rosie desexed, or spayed, and to send her ovaries and uterus to the laboratory for testing.

Joyce was very concerned by this.

'But Mr Small, she's tiny. How are you going to manage the anaesthetic? I hope she survives.'

This was a concern, but I assured Joyce that a lot of our patients were small and that we often desexed kittens and puppies for rescue agencies at an early age so that they didn't breed and contribute further to the overpopulation of cats and dogs. Joyce did not sound convinced by my reassurance, but nevertheless was happy to proceed. Besides, there was no choice for wee Rosy, we had to remove the affected tissue.

Fortunately, the surgery went well, and Rosie ended up one hundred grams lighter. She was now a mere six hundred grams!

We made sure Rosie had good aftercare and nutrition and she bounced back remarkably quickly. One of the amazing things we often find with animals is that their recovery from anaesthesia and surgical procedures is often amazingly quick, whereas the same surgery in humans can require quite prolonged recuperations. By the second day after the surgery, animals can almost be back to normal. Of course, this can lead to a false sense of security and the tendency to let a pet overdo it too early, so we often need to give strict aftercare instructions to owners. I have seen this several times myself, once when my first Burmese cat,

Lucy, or Lulu as she was affectionately known, was chasing her brother (who had also been desexed the day before) across the rooftop of our two-storey house the morning after her surgery! I had words to the owner about that to reinforce aftercare instructions.

Rosie turned out to have a granulosa cell tumour in one of her ovaries, producing hormones that were enlarging her uterus and producing her 'swollen privates'. This all settled down after she was spayed and our tiny pocket friend Rosie lived for some time after that, very happy with her new home and more comfortable in her body.

Hard of hearing

Hilda was a longstanding client of the practice and quite a character. Hilda became a customer of Courtney's in the early days when he was setting up his practice, and had been a loyal client ever since.

Hilda never married and her feline friends became her life.

Like Mrs Brown, Hilda tended to collect stray cats and look after them, and they came with their share of problems. Over the years Hilda had persuaded various handymen to build her a series of wooden extensions to the side of her house that were covered with chicken wire, allowing her to house or enclose her feline friends. She had a collection inside as well, but the less socialised fellows spent their days in these outdoor areas and could retreat to weatherproof cubbies as needed. Nowadays there would be more questions raised about the ethics of such a situation and likely some action taken.

Hilda had, over the years, become progressively harder of hearing and although she had a hearing aid fitted, it seemed to make little difference, and in fact was a health hazard to those with whom she tried to communicate due to the high-pitched screech it emitted. This was the case in both phone and face-to-face conversations with Hilda.

The phone went and I answered it. The first telltale sign that Hilda was on the phone was a long silence.

'Hello, this is Mr Small here, how can I help you?' I repeated.

Again, another silence, soon followed by a voice barking down the phone, 'Are you theeeere?'

At this stage, our suspicions were confirmed . . . it was Hilda.

'Yes, yes Hilda, it's me, Mr Small . . . how can I help you today?' I yelled at the top of my voice.

The phone handpiece had to be held twelve inches (thirty centimetres) from my ear as her hearing aid screeched down the line. It was one of those old-fashioned hearing devices that consisted of an earpiece and a handheld speaker-microphone that Hilda held at arm's length, often shoving it in your direction or frustratingly in your face, and which unpredictably and intermittently squealed and screeched at 100 decibels! This invariably caused you to recoil another metre of so if in her physical presence or hold the phone at arm's length if not.

What could be the problem today, I wondered.

After another pause Hilda started up again with her usual screeching monologue. She had obviously registered that she had made contact and it was time to proceed.

'I need you to come over. Daisy is not doing well, she's off her food and vomiting and she's quite weak.'

Now it was always difficult in a mixed practice to do house calls at the best of times as they often took quite a long time and time was in short supply. Hilda lived in the adjacent city, twelve kilometres away. But I had no choice because Hilda had no transport and Daisy needed attention.

'All right Hilda, I'll finish my morning consultations and then come over with nurse after lunch, OK?'

'What's that?' Hilda barked.

'OK, HILDA, WE WILL BE THERE THIS AFTERNOON,' I yelled.

'Good, I'll be expecting you then,' she replied.

A feeling of dread filled me as I put down the phone. Trips to Hilda's always took way longer than planned and I never felt as if I had done enough when I left nor been fully understood. The situation was always a bit surreal. Nevertheless, the cats were her life and they were well fed and cared for.

Hilda's house was in dire need of decluttering and there were boxes and newspapers stacked high in each room with paths weaving through them. The cats were perched here and there but generally on chairs and couches that were draped with blankets, sheets, and clothes. Cat litter trays peppered the house as did food and water bowls and there was an acrid odour of ammonia that permeated the air and seeped into your clothes while you were there. Oh well, Hilda was happy, and the cats appeared equally so. Surprisingly, there were few altercations between them, although Hilda did keep the most territorial or non-social ones in the enclosed runs.

When we arrived, a friend was there with Hilda, which made it easier for us, and I breathed a sigh of relief.

Daisy did not look too good and, as was often the case, I suspect Hilda had been trying some home remedies first in the days preceding my visit. Poor old Daisy was, according to Hilda, about eighteen years old, but it was difficult to tell with any certainty because she had been rescued as an adult and placed in Hilda's care.

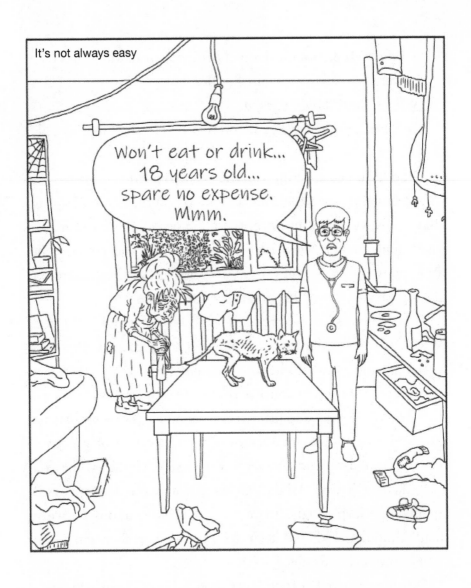

Daisy was very thin, in fact skeletal, and appeared dehydrated, as evidenced by sunken eyes and inelastic skin. She was a bit wobbly on her feet and somewhat pale. I could tell there was not a lot of hope for poor old Daisy and I asked Hilda about her recent history.

'Has she been drinking a lot of water lately, Hilda?'

'What's that?' Hilda bellowed.

Raising my voice to the high-pitched squealing and crackling receiver-speaker thrust towards my face with a brisk extension of Hilda's elbow, I repeated: 'HAS DAISY BEEN REALLY THIRSTY LATELY, HILDA?'

'Oh, there's so many of them it's difficult to tell but someone's been drinking a lot lately as the water bowls need filling more often. She's been losing weight and eating less, I know that.'

I had my suspicions that Daisy had end-stage kidney failure or diabetes. A quick look in Daisy's mouth revealed some ulcers on her gums at the back and sides of her mouth and these were infected. We managed to get a urine sample from Daisy, and it was very dilute but did not contain any glucose. This confirmed my worst fears that Daisy most likely had end-stage kidney disease and not diabetes. But how to communicate this to Hilda?

It is always a very difficult situation when you are faced with a very attached owner who has no idea how sick or advanced the disease is in their pet. One of the interesting things is that often clients do not think of their animal in the same terms as they think of themselves, with similar organs and systems, which in fact we have. It often helps to better understand the seriousness of the condition if we can imagine the grim outlook for a person who is that ill. As difficult as this is to do, we can then see the reality a little more clearly.

A blood test will normally demonstrate very high levels of kidney biochemical markers confirming the diagnosis of kidney disease.

An intravenous drip and supportive therapy can often result in some limited improvement, but it is often very temporary. However, if the disease is acute or of sudden onset and especially in a younger patient, then there is some hope. In this case we had chronic (longstanding and progressive) and acute (sudden-onset) kidney failure together with major complications and there was little hope. Any treatment was only going to result in more suffering with a poor outcome. Prolonging death, not prolonging life, in other words.

As is often the case in this sad situation, we spent some time discussing this and finally Hilda agreed that we should euthanise Daisy, or put her to sleep. This was the best course of action for Daisy and we managed to do this very peacefully.

We never take this privilege for granted and it is always very well considered. We are lucky that we have this option for our animal patients and can relieve inevitable suffering near the end or where there is no hope. Of course, we need to be very careful to communicate using the right words: euthanase or euthanise (sometimes euthanatise is used). The commonly used phrase for this procedure – put to sleep – can have a double meaning and the consequences of miscommunication would be dire.

Even though Hilda had sadly lost Daisy, she still had one or two to care for.

How old?

Not coming from a farming background, I felt some trepidation about dealing with 150-odd farmer clients. But I was not the first veterinarian to be in this position and, after all, I'd had five years of veterinary-school training, including a lot of practical work, and farmers were good sorts . . . If my vet service were of a high standard and I was friendly, there would be no worries. Right?

As it turned out my anxieties proved unfounded. Having Courtney around training me and putting in a good word for me, combined with my own youthful enthusiasm (or bravado), hard work and dedication to client satisfaction paid dividends. I had my father to thank for some of these attributes as he had a strong work ethic, sense of fairness and high moral values.

I had only been at the clinic a year or so when I had a conversation with one of my farmer clients, Jack Gunn, in the car park, after he had been in to buy some sheep vaccine and drench.

At the end of our professional conversation about animal health and the obligatory remarks about the weather, Jack looked at me inquisitively and asked, 'How old are you?'

I was a bit taken aback as normally personal questions were, if not off limits, at least not asked directly but gleaned through gossip or farmer chat sessions over the local phone or while leaning on the farm gate or back of the ute.

Anyway, I had nothing to hide so I blurted out, 'Twenty-six.'

Jack took a step back, or a stagger more like it. 'What! Bloody hell,' he exclaimed, 'I thought you were at least thirty-five and married with several kids.'

In my family we always looked a bit older than our numerical years, and in my case it may have had something to do with the familial male-pattern baldness passed down from my paternal grandfather, made worse by the stressful years at veterinary school. In this case I was pleased to appear older than my years, to some of my clients anyway, as this gave the impression of being more experienced than I was. To some people, the appearance of a fresh-faced veterinary graduate tending to their stock or beloved pet, not unreasonably, would do little to quell their sense of apprehension and anxiety. Anyway, why not take advantage of this? There had to be some bonus for premature hair loss and looking older than your years!

A barren tale

There are not many dairy farms around Napier; most of the farms run beef cattle. Black Aberdeen Angus (known simply as Angus) of Scottish origin is the predominant breed, but there are also Hereford, Charolais and Simmental.

Some large blocks ran up to a thousand head of cattle, but one to five hundred cows is more typical. Mineral deficiencies are common in Hawke's Bay and in fact throughout New Zealand, the main elements that are low in soil being copper, cobalt, selenium and occasionally iodine. The main symptoms of mineral deficiency are failure to grow or thrive, rough and light-coloured coats, and diarrhoea. Where deficiency occurs, supplementation with these minerals produces excellent results. It is amazing how calves or fawns – deer were also farmed – suddenly start to thrive, gain weight, and improve coat colour after supplementation.

I headed out with Courtney for the first few months to learn the ropes of pregnancy-testing. I had only done a few tests as part of my veterinary training and needed to upskill fast. Pregnancy-testing of cattle in those days could not be done until six weeks after a successful mating and it was easier to confirm a positive or negative from the twelve-week point. When we arrived at the farm the farmers would have the cattle in pens, or certainly enough penned to make a start. Cows were then fed into the chute and brought forward one by one to test. The veterinarian would don arm-length disposable plastic gloves and then don a calving gown, tied at the back, to protect the rest of the body. A good pair of steel-capped reasonably long boots was essential because the next step was to get in behind the cow. A lubricated and gloved arm was then inserted gently into the rectum of the cow and advanced while palpating for signs of pregnancy. You palpate for a foetus, or the amniotic sac, or cotyledons (the tuft of villi on the foetal side of the cow's placenta), amongst other things.

This job was not for the faint-hearted. It was good to be fit because it was hard work, and you often had to make your way through hundreds of cows in one day. As gentle as you tried to be, some customers were understandably not too impressed with this procedure, so it was best to quickly get in close to the cow or you might otherwise get a full-force back-hander as one or other hind leg shot back and collected your thigh. I suffered two such quad-riceps insults and the resulting haematomas left me unable to walk normally for several weeks! Twisted elbows and strained ligaments were not uncommon either, and of course quite often the sense of fullness created by your arm in the rectum resulted in an evacuation of contents, hence the need for the waterproof or poop-proof gown. In saying all this, most cows did not seem to mind at all and on a cold morning the vet definitely had the warmest job in the yard!

Now if you think this doesn't sound like a glamorous job, you would be correct. However, it is rewarding to be able to help determine whether a cow is pregnant or 'empty', as we called it. Pregnancy-testing helps with decisions such as feed management and which cows to retain or cull.

On one particular day we had driven one hour along the Napier–Taupo road to a large farm not too far from the midway point. There was a lot of forestry land along the way, mostly devoted to quick-growing radiata pine, interspersed with sheep or cattle and deer farms. The road in those days was very tortuous with lots of sharp bends and undulating hills. Along the way there were always logging trucks on the road and these were loaded up with freshly cut logs being transported to the pulp and paper mill at Whirinaki, just north of Napier. The trucks heading out from the mill moved along at a good pace but those coming back were often fully laden, so being stuck behind one made for a slow trip. The drivers were professional of course, but there was always a degree of trepidation if you were heading out to a farm and they were thundering around a corner towards you with what looked like a precarious and heavy load.

As we arrived at the farm there was the usual greeting party of farm dogs barking and escorting the car down to the yards. There was always the worry you might run over one, but they were very adept at keeping out of the way, thankfully.

As I looked at the yards I could not help but notice there was quite an assembled mass of cows. This was going to be some days' work!

Walt, the farm manager, was standing by the yard as we pulled up. A grunt of acknowledgement was followed by a brief how-do. Walt was a man of few words and his weathered and ruddy complexion reflected his years in the saddle battling the elements on the farm. The winters up here were pretty harsh, often bitterly cold with howling winds and a frequent dusting of snow. The summers could be very dry with long sun-filled days, although never too warm, and there was often a cool breeze.

I was amazed at Courtney's stamina, given he was now on the other side of sixty. There must have been five to six hundred cows in front of us in need of a yeah-or-nay diagnosis today.

So, off we went with me stepping in to do a few as we went along. I could see this was an efficient team and a steady stream of customers was presented one after the other for testing. As we progressed, it appeared there was a good pregnancy rate with not many dry cows (non-pregnant).

Then it was my turn again and I was pleased that the going was relatively easy and there was only the odd tricky diagnosis. But I was having trouble with one cow. She seemed a bit more rattled or edgy compared to most of the other cows we'd seen. As I removed my left arm and inserted my right arm, thinking I might get a better feel, the cow thrust her rear end from left to right and gave my elbow a good wrench. This was not the place to complain, though, and after a while the discomfort settled. I noticed the yard had gone quiet, apart from the odd murmur and chuckle. I was still having trouble and was just about to make a judgement call after what seemed an uncomfortably long period, when Walt piped up. 'You'll have trouble calling that one young vet.'

With those ominous words the penny dropped.

Sure enough, as the assembled workers erupted in laughter, I glanced down to see that my customer was in fact a steer not a cow. The rotten buggers, I thought. I'll bet that's not the first time they've done that. Of course, to the initiated, the rear end of a steer looks quite different to that of a cow. I should have known.

I had a laugh as well, but I had learnt my lesson. If there are tricky ones, and a farmer is involved, keep your wits about you and check the sex!

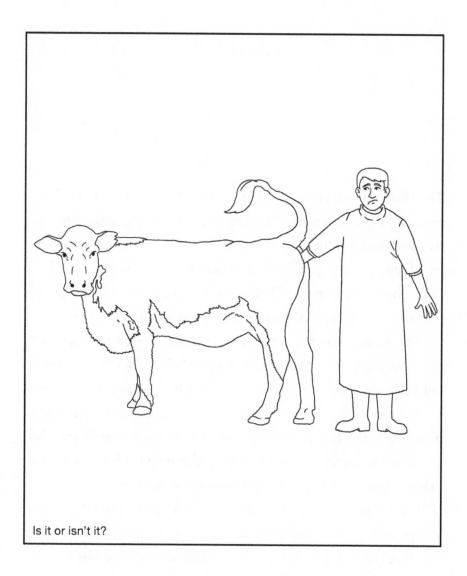

Is it or isn't it?

Glass full

The Watsons ran an up-market country lodge with a fine-dining restaurant and accommodation on site. The grounds were impressive and exquisitely manicured with exotic plantings. Outdoor weddings, garden parties and functions of all sorts were held throughout the season. There was a wonderful old two-storey homestead with formal entertaining rooms and a ballroom.

The Watsons were always immaculately dressed and were real characters with larger-than-life personalities. They drove stately old Mercedes cars and knew how to love life and live it to the full.

We received an invitation to dinner one night to celebrate a birthday. I had heard stories about the culinary skill of the chef and that the menu was fine French and top end. This would be a Friday night to enjoy, I thought, a rare indulgence.

I did have to work that weekend but that was OK, I was young, and anyway we would leave in good time.

We arrived and were immediately greeted like long-lost friends, ushered straight in, and given a glass of fine French champagne and offered hors d'oeuvres. As we sank into the sumptuous chaise longues I could not help thinking that this was a different world compared to my work the day before. No, no, there would be no talk of pregnancy-testing tonight.

As we reclined and sipped the expensive bubbly, I mused about how vastly different people's lifestyles could be, but was happy with my lot. I did enjoy the rural work and the down-to-earth friendly farmers I worked with. Besides, that was what I had trained for and I was going to make the most of it.

The pianist had a good repertoire and we relaxed and listened.

Eventually we were seated for our meal and by this stage I had sampled a fine Belgian beer followed by a Japanese Sapporo beer. As we sat down, I could not help but notice the line-up of glasses in front of each place setting. Admittedly, one of them was a water glass, but there was also a champagne glass, a beer glass, a white-wine glass, a red-wine glass and what looked like a sherry or maybe liqueur glass, for each diner. There were a collection of what looked like fine wines, both red and white, at the other end of the table. Mr Watson proceeded to run through the selection explaining the country of origin, winemaking region, vintage and finally the rather expensive price of each wine before removing the cork and pouring a glass of each into the assembled glasses. By this stage, my inhibitions were somewhat lowered and with the host's hospitality and expertise as he expounded on the virtues of each wine, who could refuse! I had never seen such an expensive line-up.

As the evening went on and each tasty and exquisitely presented dish appeared, the level of wine in the glasses in front of me never seemed to fall below full. The beer, champagne, white- and red-wine glasses were being topped up as soon as a mouthful was taken, and I had only just realised it. Everything was starting to become a little hazy by then and at the end of the meal I seem to remember trying a selection of different liqueurs to finish off the meal, accompanied by some fine chocolates. The storytelling grew wilder and wilder, the words thicker and thicker and one thing seemed to blend into another.

As it came time to depart I felt a pang of regret or perhaps trepidation, but by this stage I was long past worrying. As I stood up there was a vague sense of malaise, and the room began spinning, but I managed to steady myself and make some sort of fitting statement, uttering my profound thanks for a most memorable evening. At least that is what I thought I said, but I was not in any state to know.

Luckily, we had transport home. I can remember the room spinning a fair bit once I was home and I tried not to think of the morning to come.

As expected, the next day was not an easy one and between my appointments my amused receptionist knew where to find me when the next client arrived – out the back door, lying on the wooden ramp with my eyes closed, resting in the cool breeze. Fortunately, it was not a busy day. Understandably I was not offered a lot of sympathy, rather, I appeared to be the source of a general amusement. It was the second day in a row I was providing others with amusement and on this occasion I only had myself to blame.

A stab in the dark

Brett was a good farmer. He had migrated from Australia where the weather conditions in his area were becoming increasingly dry and harsh, making farming difficult. He was pleased with the family's move and had settled in well, running a sheep and cattle farm and doing some bull breeding on the side. His aim was to improve the quality of his stock and offer premium bulls of high genetic merit, resulting in progeny with fast growth rates and increased bodyweights. This involved artificial insemination with imported semen.

This produced valuable offspring. Breeding dates had to be carefully recorded so pregnancy could be monitored, feeding optimised and calving dates predicted. Any difficulty with calving meant early intervention because the calf and cow were valuable.

The phone rang at two in the morning. I turned over, picked it up and muttered, 'Hello.'

'Is that Mike?'

'Yes, it's Mike here,' I replied.

'It's Brett Robertson here, Mike. One of my cows, Mary, is having difficulty calving and I need you to come out now.'

'OK,' I replied, 'I'll get dressed and be on my way. I'll see you in about an hour.'

I scrambled to the clinic and loaded up the necessary gear, expecting that a field caesarean might be necessary. It was always a challenge to make sure that you never forgot anything as it was a long way back to the clinic to collect an important piece of equipment and time was of the essence.

Now Windermere was about three-quarters of an hour's drive directly west of Napier on a winding undulating road. I made good time as the road was deserted, unsurprisingly.

When I arrived we loaded up the tractor with my equipment before heading out to the paddock where our patient was sitting down. She was in second-stage labour and Brett had tried to assist her with a natural birth, but it appeared there was not enough room in the pelvis to allow the calf to be born. I put on a glove and lubricant and confirmed Brett's assessment. The calf was alive – I could feel it moving as I was doing the examination.

'Well, Brett, the calf is still alive so that's great news, but we are going to have to do a caesarean I am afraid.'

'I thought as much,' he replied.

So, I administered some dissociative anaesthesia and pain relief, and infiltrated the surgical site on Mary's side with local anaesthetic. While I was waiting for the drugs to work, I laid out my kit on a large sterile drape in the paddock. We were working under the lights of the tractor and a cold wind was blowing. I was keen to scrub my hands clean and wash them with the warm water Brett had provided. It was not going to be so bad for me as I would be working for some of the time inside the warm patient, although she would not have had the same feelings I suspected!

Everything that you are taught never prepares you for an emergency caesarean in the middle of the night with a cold wind blowing working under the lights of a farm tractor in the middle of an often muddy paddock.

But there was an important job to be done and that was my focus.

Brett, of course, was my able-bodied assistant.

It was not long before we had the calf out. Brett managed to help lift her free, give her a rub down and make sure she was breathing after clearing her mouth of mucous. The calf was stable, so Brett returned to assist me with the sewing up.

At this point, despite spending time removing the calf from the warm cow, I was starting to feel a bit of wind chill and, given it was about four in the morning by then, maybe a little light-headed. I had used a scalpel to make the incisions in Mary's side and to cut down through the layers of the body wall and into the uterus to remove the calf. The handiest place to hold the scalpel when not in use was between my teeth. Now this was not text-book nor particularly conventional, but the lighting was dim, and I wanted to have it handy as I needed to extend the length of my incision a couple of times.

I was preoccupied with getting ready to sew up Mary and had momentarily forgotten about the scalpel in my mouth. Brett had come back and was helping to hold the tissues up for me with gloved hands as I started to sew.

At that point Brett asked me a question and as I started to reply the scalpel made a downward dive, as the laws of gravity dictate, and lodged in Brett's forearm, coming to an abrupt stop, upright, when the tip contacted his ulna! Without a blink or a sound Brett took the handle of the scalpel in his other hand and pulled it out of his arm and laid it to one side with the rest of the surgical kit.

Uttering profound apologies, I hurriedly returned to the patient to complete the suturing.

To my surprise Brett did not want me to sew up the neat incision in his arm. Fortunately, there was little bleeding and the wound was small. Nevertheless, it must have hurt. I never did that again!

A sour affair

Ralph was a big rough-coated dog. He weighed about thirty-eight kilograms and like many of my canine patients he was of hybrid pedigree, or in common speak – a mongrel, bitzer or mutt. Mongrel or mutt have taken on more derogatory meanings in recent times, so a nicer way to describe his breed pedigree would be mixed-breed. Ralph was certainly big and strong – or he was usually!

On this day, Ralph was sitting in the waiting room looking depressed and lethargic. His third eyelids, or haws, the protective inner membrane that can move across the eye to protect it from injury or insult, were partially prolapsed, sitting across the inner surface of his eyes. He had strings of saliva, or drool, hanging from the sides of his mouth.

I motioned to Rob to bring Ralph into the consulting room for an examination.

'Good morning, Rob. I see Ralph isn't looking too good today. What's the story?'

'No, Doc, he's pretty poorly. He ain't eaten his tucker for two days and he's lyin' around more than usual.'

'That's no good. Is he showing any other clinical signs of illness?' I asked.

'Well, Doc, he's drooling a lot and he's retching a bit. Can't hold anything down. He's making a real mess. Haven't seen any poop for a couple of days. He ain't right, no doubt about that.'

I examined Ralph and he appeared dehydrated with slightly sunken eyes. His gum colour was not its usual pink but a muddy colour and the capillary refill (how quickly the colour returns to his gums when you press on them for a second then release your finger), was slow. His tummy felt empty but was not painful. I listened to his chest and the lung sounds were somewhat raspy and his breathing rate elevated. Ralph's temperature was normal.

'Has he eaten anything unusual that you know of Rob?'

'Nup, not that I know of, Doc, but he's always chewin' on things he shouldn't, or on the scrounge for what he can get – it often comes out the backend, if it stays down that is.'

Mmm, I thought, that's interesting.

'Rob, we better keep him in and put him on a drip, check his bloods and take X-rays to see if we can work out what the problem is, OK?'

'Whatever you say, Doc. We just want him right.'

I could see Ralph was not well at all and it was difficult to know what was going on without further investigation but it looked like there might be some sort of upper gastrointestinal tract problem as he was drooling and couldn't hold down any food or fluid. He was off his food too, which was highly unusual.

So, we admitted Ralph, took a blood sample, put him on an intravenous drip and treated his symptoms. We also administered drugs to help relieve his discomfort and drooling and fluids to rehydrate him.

The blood test did not show anything remarkable, but he had an elevated white blood-cell count which could mean infection or inflammation and his red blood-cell count and blood protein were increased a little, probably due to dehydration.

The next step was to get an X-ray of Ralph's chest to have a look at his heart, lungs and his oesophagus, as it passes through his chest on the way to the stomach.

Ralph was a big boy, but he was co-operative, and we managed to get two X-rays – one with him lying on his left side and the other on his right. We had to process X-ray film in a dark room just like a photo studio at home. You took the film from the cassette in a dark room and developed it in a developer solution, rinsed it in water, then fixed it in a fixer solution before finally rinsing it and hanging it to dry. Of course, nowadays we have digital radiography where an image is taken and processed without the need for X-ray developing chemicals. The X-ray cassette, which the image is projected onto when the picture is taken, is placed in an automatic processor and the image is developed digitally. Back then we had a slower and messier process with potentially toxic chemicals, so today's technology is most welcome, allowing you also to enhance the image for better viewing and interpretation.

As I held the image up to the red light in the dark room a degree of unease came over me. What was that? I thought. Bang smack in the oesophagus just in front of the heart shadow in the chest was a large ovoid object that should not have been there! Normally the oesophagus appeared as a thin collapsed tube that could be hard to see on the X-ray, although often there might be some gas in it which appears as a thin black shadow. What I was seeing today was far from normal. My heart skipped a few beats thinking about the options here.

Once the X-ray film was fixed, I rinsed it and took it through to the X-ray viewer box (a backlit box on the wall for viewing X-rays).

'Rob, can you see that on the X-ray film?' I said, pointing to the ovoid object in the chest. 'That should not be there and indicates a foreign body in Ralph's oesophagus.'

Rob muttered a few expletives, then he confirmed my suspicions. 'It looks like one of those bloody lemons from the lemon tree in the backyard that he likes chewing on.'

I could only agree unfortunately! 'It does, Rob. I thought it looked like a lemon. Does he really normally chew on lemons?'

'Yep, he loves them and normally chews them up as they fall, but he's been known to jump up and steal them right off the tree.'

I was surprised that a dog would eat something so acidic, but as the years rolled on, I realised that virtually nothing is off limits for some of our canine companions. If it was food of any kind, it could be eaten. If it smells – preferably the smellier the better – and if there is any possibility it can be swallowed, then it generally is. If it can't be swallowed it might be licked; failing that, it was good to roll in! The world out there is a cocktail of great aromas and gustatory opportunities for many of our canine friends. Why Ralph had swallowed the lemon whole this time I couldn't explain!

'Well, Rob, we are going to have to open up Ralph's chest and remove that lemon. It's pretty big and it's not going anywhere on its own. The surgery's a bit risky so we will need to stabilise him first, then operate.'

'Well, Doc, I trust you and it looks like we have no choice.'

I agreed and Rob went home to share the unusual story with his wife and await my call.

In those days it was not unusual to have to do a thoracotomy – open up the chest cavity – to surgically solve a problem. Nowadays, referral to a specialist for non-invasive laparoscopic surgery or to perform a thoracotomy is more common.

Finances were an issue for Rob and whatever I was to do for Ralph had to be on time payment. But our immediate concern was Ralph. So, we set about removing the lemon.

Once Ralph's chest cavity was open, Debbie, my nurse, performed intermittent positive pressure ventilation (IPPV), to breathe for Ralph. Once the chest is entered the negative pressure gradient is removed and the patient cannot breathe adequately for themselves. IPPV is relatively easy to do but needs just enough pressure to inflate the lungs, maintain good oxygenation and allow the heart to refill with blood between breaths. So, I surgically removed the lemon from the distended oesophagus and then sutured the oesophagus and chest cavity closed. We instilled long-acting local anaesthetic around the rib area and gave Ralph antibiotics and strong pain relief. He was only to have water and liquid food in small amounts after a day or two. Surprisingly, Ralph recovered well but unfortunately it was not good news for the lemon tree. By the time Ralph went home it was a lemon tree no more, which was probably for the best as Ralph may not have survived another operation . . . or so I thought.

Too close to call

It was several years later when the phone rang, and it was Rob.

'Is that Dr Mike?' he asked.

'It is,' I replied.

'It's Rob here, Ralph's owner. Do you remember us?'

Well now, that was a fair question, I thought, but how could I forget?

If there is one thing for sure it is that once you have seen a patient for a major problem and spoken to an owner a few times, there is no way that you are going to forget them, ever! Often, even if you cannot remember the whole story, the association of the owner's name and the animal's name triggers instant recall. And if they suddenly appear in the waiting room, even if it's many years later, generally there is instant recognition.

'How could I forget! How is Ralph?'

I knew with certainty that was a question that wasn't going to have a 'He's fine, Doc,' answer, as Rob wasn't inclined to ring me for small talk or to pass the time of day.

'He's not too good, Doc. He's just lyin' on the back concrete path and he won't budge. Can't move him. Can you come over?'

That does not sound good, I thought. Rob didn't live far away and the quickest thing was to drive over and assess the situation.

'OK, Rob, I'll be over in ten minutes.'

When I arrived with Debbie, my nurse, there was Ralph prostrate on the concrete on his side and not looking good at all. There was no lemon tree in sight!

'How long has he been lying here, Rob?' I asked.

'Just found him now, Doc.'

'And no lemons to blame. What's been happening the last day or two, Rob?' I asked.

'Well, he's been out of sorts and then yesterday he seemed real dopey like and wouldn't eat.'

'Anything else?' I asked.

'Nope,' he replied.

Now, it's interesting that often there are not many obvious symptoms of illness, but sometimes people just don't notice things. Some owners are very observant and notice any little change in their animal's behaviour. Others just go about their lives and for one reason or other aren't particularly observant, or in some cases are too busy, or worse, neglectful, to pay enough attention to their animals. Often people do not think of their pets as they think of themselves, so alarm bells can be slow to ring.

In Rob's case I think he was just not very observant until there was obviously a major problem.

I thought that Ralph's abdomen looked swollen, so I asked Rob about this.

'Have you noticed his belly's swollen, Rob?'

'Now you come to mention it, yeah it does look a bit bloated,' he replied.

I was not sure what the cause was, but I knew it wasn't good.

Ralph's mucous membrane colour (in this case his gum colour) was good. In fact, it was too good and the cherry red suggested congestion. He was breathing very quickly in short shallow breaths and obviously in a lot of discomfort.

'It's not looking very good, Rob,' I remarked, quickly feeling like I was stating the obvious. 'We need to transport him straight back to the clinic to see what's going on.'

We loaded Ralph onto a stretcher and carried him to the back of the station wagon and hurried him back to the surgery.

I took an X-ray and all we could see was a big whitish abdomen with a lack of detail. Better see what is in that abdomen, I thought, so I inserted a fine needle and drew out some fluid. It was a very light-coloured clear fluid with a slight yellow tinge and smelt remarkably like urine.

My heart sank as I realised that I hadn't tapped urine from Ralph's bladder; it had come directly from his abdominal cavity where it should not be. It must have come from a ruptured structure, most likely the bladder.

I attempted to pass a urinary catheter up Ralph's urethra, and it would only go in a short distance before it hit a dead end. Interestingly the dog's penis has a bone – os penis –along part of the mid-section. The penis of most mammalian species has an os penis, or baculum, to help maintain an erection. This leads to the mildly humorous line: 'The human penis is a puzzler, no bones about it.'

What happens in dogs is that small bladder stones, which can sometimes form in the bladder over time, especially in some breeds, pass down the urethra or urine tube and lodge behind the beginning of the os penis, which almost completely surrounds the urethra in this area. This results in the partial or complete inability to urinate and creates a lot of discomfort for the dog. It can quickly become life-threatening. We normally see the patient in the early to mid-stages of a partial or complete blockage, before the bladder fills so much that it ruptures. Not so today.

Who would have believed that Ralph would have another major problem of such severity? But you know the old saying: It never rains but it pours. True in Ralph's case.

I did not like Ralph's chances.

I picked up the phone and dialled Rob's number.

'Rob, it's not looking good. Ralph has a ruptured bladder because his urethra has become blocked by bladder stones, so he hasn't been able to urinate. It's very serious, he will need emergency surgery once I have stabilised him, but it is very risky. What do you want me to do?'

'Hell, Doc, that sounds real bad. There's no way we can lose Ralph, he's one of the family.'

My heart sank again. I didn't rate Ralph's chances of a recovery very high.

But I said, 'I'll do my best, Rob, leave it with me.'

With that I hung up the phone and we set to work.

Ralph's bloods were not too bad, with his kidney markers elevated moderately and electrolytes slightly abnormal, as expected. But they could have been a lot worse. We started him on fluids and shortly after gave him some anaesthetic with great care.

When we opened Ralph's abdominal cavity we had to have plenty of towels under him and good suction to remove the large amount of urine that had accumulated. We flushed his abdominal cavity with lots of saline, as urine can be quite damaging to other organs. It was hard to believe that Ralph's bladder was as ruptured as it was, the length of the tear ran from right in his pelvic area to the other end, or front of his bladder. I could barely see the back, or caudal, torn end of the bladder as it ran into his pelvic area. I checked for any bladder stones floating in the abdomen and we found a few which we flushed out with saline. I managed to suture the bladder, but it was a big job and the resulting line of sutures was very long. Luckily, the bladder and abdominal organs looked OK otherwise, despite the irritant effects of urine in the abdomen.

I had attempted to flush the stones lodged in the urethra back into the bladder before I closed it, to clear the blockage, but they would not budge. There was no choice then but to cut down over the area and remove them through the opening I created. Luckily, this was possible as the bone did not go all the way around the urethra but was open along the underside.

I cut down and removed two stones that were definitely not going to budge. How they got there in the first place is always a mystery but most likely when the animal urinates the urethra dilates with the fluid and it gives them more of a chance to migrate to this position.

We leave the bottom of this cut open to heal naturally and although the animal pees or urinates through this hole for a period, it generally closes over quickly, and they resume urinating from the end of the penis before long.

To my great surprise Ralph was very stable throughout the surgery and made a good recovery.

It always fascinates me that when you suture up the bladder it can still fill and empty without rupturing again during the healing phase. We try to get clients to take their pets out frequently to toilet, so it doesn't fill up too much and strain the bladder sutures. I have never had to re-suture a bladder after this sort of surgery, which is quite amazing when you think about it.

Ralph made an amazing recovery and within a day or two his kidney markers were back to normal and he was back to his happy and ravenous self. What was even more amazing was that he was thirteen years old by then!

He was a tough cookie and fortunately for Ralph, and Rob's pocket, we were not to see that tough old dog again for anything major during his lifetime.

Slip sliding away

Since European settlement in New Zealand, there have been wild deer and pigs in many parts of the country and hunting has become a common pastime. Within easy reach of Napier are mountain ranges and forestry blocks, particularly in close proximity to the Napier–Taupo Highway, so the hunting is often good.

Pig dogs are used to assist in the hunt. The wild boars that are being pursued, when cornered, can inflict some impressive wounds on the dog and usually require veterinary attention. I soon accepted that pig-dog hunting is a reality and our role as vets is to provide veterinary services where needed.

Des was a recreational pig hunter and he had several dogs that he trained for this purpose. One Saturday afternoon Des had just got back from a forestry block where he had been hunting with his dogs. Gyp had tracked a large boar and cornered it, whereupon it had turned on him and lashed out, inflicting nasty wounds around his neck area and on his side.

Around four, Des phoned from the clinic car park.

'Hi, Doc, I got Gyp in my car and he needs some stitches, he's been stuck by a boar.'

I had not long been home from the Saturday morning clinic but luckily had had a late lunch and a break, so it wasn't a bad time to call.

'I'll be down in ten minutes, just wait there Des.' I said. When I got to the clinic, there was the usual 4WD SUV vehicle with bull bars and roof rack to hold the catch. Des and Gyp were inside and a more senior gentleman was sitting in the passenger seat.

'Come on in and let's have a look.'

Gyp certainly had been stuck by the boar and there were some deep puncture wounds around his neck, luckily not involving any major structures, and a gash on his neck. The jugular vein and carotid arteries run up and down each side of the neck and thankfully these were unharmed. Sometimes if the tusk enters the chest cavity it is very serious indeed, but Gyp's breathing seemed quite regular and settled, so this was unlikely.

'I am going to have to give Gyp an anaesthetic and clip, clean and suture the wounds Des,' I announced.

'I thought as much,' Des replied.

'OK, leave him with me and I'll call you when he's ready.'

'Hey, Doc, I really want to stay with Gyp. He's my best mate you know. I want to be with him while you sew him up,' Des announced.

Now this was always tricky. I preferred the client not be present during the anaesthetic, for good reason. It was often a distraction and keeping an eye on the patient as well as the owner who is standing in the room is a bit much to ask, especially in the midst of a surgical task.

But Des was insistent and wasn't going to take no for an answer. His father seemed to support this position. He had one arm in a sling, having just undergone surgery himself for a shoulder injury, and was looking a bit dishevelled with wiry white hair and an impressive stubble overlying a weather-beaten face. I suspect Dad had been, or still was, a pig hunter as well and had spent some time in the elements. Des was a slight, wiry man like his father, wearing the trademark Swanndri jacket, boots, and shorts. Swanndri is an outdoor clothing company from New Zealand. I wondered how he lugged the dead pig back to the vehicle given his size, but these characters were often amazingly tough and deceptively strong.

'OK, Des. I don't normally allow clients in the surgery for all sorts of reasons, but just this once I'll make an exception.' It was Saturday afternoon and he was used to blood and wounds for sure, so I thought it should be OK.

In those days, without a nurse available, Des could give me a hand while I anaesthetised Gyp. Once Gyp was out to it, I clipped the wounds and cleaned them with antiseptic solution and laid out the surgical kit.

As I opened the wounds and removed the embedded hair and debris to enable me to flush and clean them before suturing the deep tears, all appeared to be going well. Des and his father were standing to my right at the end of the table with their backs to the wall. It was a small room with the afternoon sun shining through the window as it descended in the sky. I was focused on the job at hand, but was mindful of my onlookers. Often hunters were men of few words and Des was no exception, so I wasn't too fazed by the silence in the room.

There were a few bleeders as I trimmed the tissue and I soon had them clamped and ligated. It was getting a bit warm in the room with four of us in there, including Gyp.

98

Out of the corner of my right eye I spotted a slight movement from Des's direction. I turned to see Des slowly sliding down the wall with his feet and legs moving towards me as they slid out along the floor. It was like a slow-motion movie coming to a stop as his buttocks hit the ground and his limp upper body slumped forward. His father was no help, with the arm on Des's side in a sling and penned in as he was by the end of the surgical table. I downed my instruments and moved to prop up the white-faced Des. It was a while before Des came around. I suspect he must have had an early start that day, with little decent nourishment, as his colour was ghost white and he didn't seem too warm. Well, this is great, I thought, I've now got at least two patients and possibly three. Des's father wasn't looking too chipper by this stage either. With Des propped up against the wall and some blankets over him and a glass of water in hand, I returned to Gyp and completed the suturing.

By the time I had finished, Des was sitting a bit more upright, but still wasn't completely with it.

Gyp soon recovered and I administered some antibiotic and pain relief. They were keen to be on their way as they lived some distance from town, and it was getting late by then. I wondered whether it might be better to stay a while and recover, but they were insistent – they were fine.

Des was in no state yet to drive the car. His father with one arm in a sling wasn't much better either and Gyp wasn't any use in that regard.

So, with a recovering Gyp laid out on the back seat amidst the day's trappings, a pallid dozy Des in the passenger seat, a one-armed geriatric in the driver's seat, and a wild boar strapped to the roof rack, the insistent and ailing trio set out on the long journey home ... in a manual car! I can still see the three of them to this day, imprinted on my mind, as they left the car park: a very sorry sight, but all of them as tough and resilient as old boots. They made it home safely, thank goodness.

A wild fare

I have attended to many pig-dog wounds over the years and almost without exception the dogs themselves are some of the friendliest, most well-mannered, and obedient patients I have seen. Their owners are also generally very courteous and appreciative of my services.

Sometimes there was pressure to dispense extra suture materials and antibiotics to enable back-country treatment. However, generally the patient needs to be seen to evaluate the extent of the wounds and a veterinary decision made as to whether they need a full general anaesthetic to suture their large wounds, or just local anaesthetic to suture smaller wounds. Antibiotics, along with pain relief, are often needed as the wild boars' tusks can inflict deep wounds.

Although Des was an infrequent customer, he was normally able to pay. Not everyone was flush with money, though, and often a trade was proposed. What could be better than a quarter, or better a half, of freshly caught pig!

Doug turned up with Boris one chilly Sunday afternoon.

Boris had more extensive wounds than Gyp. He had an injury

to his jugular vein in his neck and although there had been some bleeding, that had now stopped, leaving a large blood clot in his neck. He had also suffered a penetrating wound to his chest, and I was worried that he could develop a chest infection or, just as bad, what we call a pneumothorax, where air leaks from the outside into the chest cavity through the wound. However, his breathing did not appear laboured. Boris was taking it all in his stride and was obviously as tough as old boots. I administered the usual antibiotic and pain relief.

Doug took me aside to have a word in my ear.

'Look, Doc, I ain't very flush at the moment but I can offer you a side of pork as payment. It's good meat and just freshly caught. It's tasty stuff, you'll love it, Doc.'

Oooh, this is a bit difficult, I thought. I wasn't a big meat eater and wasn't sure about wild boar meat either.

Oh well, what's the harm? I thought. Besides, Boris needed attention.

'All right,' I said.

Boris's surgery went well and although the tusk had penetrated the chest cavity, I was able to suture the puncture injury closed to reseal the chest, and clean and suture his neck wound.

After the surgery I was paid with the side of pork as negotiated. Even Wesley the dog wouldn't eat it – too gamey by far. I decided wild pig meat was definitely an acquired taste, and best left to appreciative and seasoned taste buds. In future I politely declined!

Soup for lunch?

Lake Tutira is a picturesque lake north of Napier on the way to Wairoa. It is a wildlife refuge that's popular for camping and picnics. Around its edge are weeping willows and prolific bird life. The lake was declared a bird sanctuary in 1929 at the instigation of Scottish farmer, author, and ornithologist William Guthrie-Smith, who once farmed neighbouring Tutira Station. Birdlife at the lake includes scaup, grey ducks, black swans, little white-throated shags, black shags, white-faced herons, pukeko (Australasian swamphens), fantails, New Zealand wood pigeons, swallows, kingfishers – and many more. For centuries Māori seasonally lived by Lake Tutira and you can see the remains of six pa sites.

The lake has battled with overgrowth of weeds and eutrophication due to fertiliser run-off from surrounding farms. The fact that it has mainly one inlet and poor outflow doesn't help either.

Not far from the lake, but inland and higher up, Ted and Joan Buxford had been managers of Tutira Estate for twenty years or so. The estate is a remote, sprawling, hilly sheep and cattle farm which, like much of the surrounding country, is deficient in minerals. Supplementation with the elements copper, cobalt and selenium is necessary to ensure good growth in livestock.

Ted was an old-school farmer and a man of few words, but very considered and straight to the point when he did have something to say. You knew if Ted barked at you that you had better listen and act, because he meant it. Perhaps there was some army training in there somewhere, but he wasn't one to mince words. He was ruddy faced and always kitted out in oilskins unless there were clear skies, his appearance presumably the result of many years of being exposed to the harsh climate of the back country. His leather cowboy hat always firmly planted on his head, he had a dry sense of humour, and humour at someone else's expense was his favourite. Veterinarians were not exempt!

I had organised a day of pregnancy-testing and headed up there early, as there were many head of cattle to examine.

The yards for pregnancy-testing were somewhat remote from the farmhouse and over a rough hilly track so Ted gave me a ride on the back of the tractor. I had not brought any lunch as Joan had kindly insisted she would prepare a meal for us after the pregnancy-testing. We arrived at the yards about mid-morning and there was a fair-sized gathering of black steamy heads waiting in the pens and surrounding paddocks.

It wasn't long before we got underway and with my arms double gloved and five litres of lubricant at hand I was pleased to be inserting them into the depths of the warm cows on such a bitterly cold day with a chilly easterly blowing across the yards. On a day like that, movement was essential, or you might freeze on the spot.

I was making reasonable progress but I could see it was going to be mid-afternoon before we got the job done.

There were no smoko or tea breaks, so by the time we finally got to the end of the testing it was, as I'd estimated, mid-afternoon. Normally I was quite robust, but today the biting cold wind and the long line-up of candidates tested my stamina, and a smoko break would have been welcome. I hoped the late lunch was going to be good.

So, we headed back over the hill to the farmhouse, all at Ted's pace. Afterall, the vet charged by the head, not the hour!

Joan was waiting for us and after I washed and attempted to make myself as presentable as possible – not easy after dealing with four to five hundred cows, I headed inside.

Something smelt good and Joan was just finishing off the meal. I could see home-reared bacon, sausages and eggs in the pan and fried potatoes as well. There was a fresh loaf of white bread and butter on the table, and a big pot of tea. I couldn't wait to tuck in.

As we talked about the day's events Joan carefully loaded up the large soup plates with the lunch. I noticed the pan was large and deep and contained a lot of clear liquid. Probably a clear soup, I thought, which would be welcome.

As the plates were lowered to the table Ted reached over and grabbed a couple of thick slabs of bread and dunked one of them into the liquid that filled the soup bowl and started his meal. This looked good, so I followed suit.

It wasn't till I raised the sodden bread to my mouth that I realised the liquid was in fact lard, or tallow. And there was plenty of it. I chewed and swallowed the first mouthful and it was tasty enough.

Ted and Joan tucked into the meal and after eating all the fried food, they wiped their bowls clean with the last of the white bread to make sure none of the dripping was wasted. I managed to enjoy the tasty fried food but left most of the 'soup' to set, which most likely was frowned upon. 'Bloody townies,' they probably said, although too polite to say it to my face. I could feel my arteries seizing up with tallow on the drive back to town!

A rocky ride

Sam was the archetypal labrador. His coat was golden rather than the equally common black, and he had the ideal conformation for a sport or working dog, with a typical happy-go-lucky attitude. Labradors make ideal family pets and very rarely exhibit any aggressive or misdirected behaviours, are very happy to be tugged and pulled about, or to run around with young ones.

Labradors' appetites and their ability to overindulge if given half a chance are legendary. Anything and everything that can be swallowed or that remotely resembles food can be fair game and it doesn't take much to pass the labrador taste test. I can recall Rover, who regularly ate himself to a bout of diarrhoea on fallen plums, or Sally, who made a daily ritual of vacuuming and chewing up all the fallen lemons, like the unfortunate Ralph. I had one client who used to feed his labrador whole chicken carcasses and I never had to operate for an obstruction – sheer luck I would say. That is something we don't recommend for a whole variety of reasons! Labradors may have an amazing digestive tract, but nevertheless they can only handle so much before intervention is needed.

Bert Goldsack looked a little concerned as he waited to be seen with Sam, who wasn't his usual energetic and boisterous self.

As Bert walked Sam into the examination room he recounted some history.

'Well, Doc, lately he's not been eating much, which is not like Sam. He's not losing weight though. In fact, he looks like he's gaining it – his stomach has got bigger.'

As I looked at Sam I noticed that he did look a little like a sow that was ready to farrow or an expectant bitch, but Sam was a neutered male!

'Oh yeah, Doc, and when he walks he rattles. It stops when he stops walking though.'

That is unusual, I thought. As Sam walked into the consulting room, I could hear a clicking and clacking sound that appeared to be coming from Sam! On the surface it was quite comical, but to the vet in me, concerning.

'Thanks Bert, I'll just see what I can find.'

I knelt down to examine Sam. A quick examination confirmed my suspicions. When I pushed up on the underside of Sam's belly, I could hear a sound exactly like river stones clicking and clacking along the bottom of a briskly flowing river, and I could feel small weights shifting under my hand, exactly like stones!

'Bert, this might seem like a strange question but has Sam been eating stones?'

'Well, funny you should mention that, Doc. Now the weather has been better we have been heading to the beach a lot more. He likes to run after the stones we throw and skim along the water,' Bert volunteered.

What better way to exercise Sam and while away the beach

walk than to skip flat stones along the water's edge with Sam in hot pursuit. Sam obviously thought this was great fun and spent many a happy hour chasing stones.

'It looks like he's swallowing some of them. We had better take an X-ray and see if that is what has happened,' I said.

An X-ray confirmed our suspicions – multiple flat reasonably sized river stones filled Sam's stomach. Poor Sam.

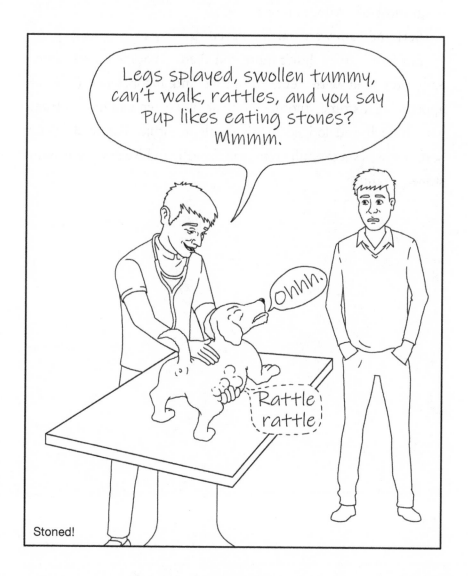

Stoned!

I showed Bert the X-ray and explained what we needed to do.

'Well, Bert, there is only one way to treat Sam today. We need to anaesthetise him for a gastrostomy – open his stomach – and remove the stones. He'll be a new dog afterwards and his appetite will return for sure.'

The outcome was indeed all good news for Sam. A successful gastrostomy removed ten large beach stones with a resultant weight loss of a kilogram or more.

Bert and Sam were much relieved.

But Sam's story didn't quite end there . . . Some months later Sam presented with acute vomiting and inappetence (lack of appetite). This time, another stone he had eaten had moved from his stomach and lodged in his small intestine. Fortunately for Sam this was successfully removed as well, and we never saw Sam stoned again!

Food fest

Dogs are carnivores and have relatively short digestive tracts so they need easily digestible, high-quality diets. The stomach acidity in dogs is much lower than in humans and this may be one of the reasons why they are less affected by 'garbage gastritis' than us (stomach upsets caused by eating the wrong or unsavoury food). However, overall, their digestive tract and in fact their whole body system is not too dissimilar to ours.

It is relatively easy for a veterinarian to understand body systems as that is what we have studied. Sometimes, despite our best intentions, we see our patients later, rather than sooner. This can happen for a variety of reasons. Animals are quite good at masking their symptoms, at least for a time, and this may be related to the phenomenon of survival of the fittest, or survival in the wild. There is no survival advantage to falling victim to an illness in the wild. Often, too, in the busyness of life, a pet's early symptoms of illness may go unnoticed. The other reason is that not everyone compares an animal, or their pet, to themselves. I often ask clients to think of their pets exactly as they would themselves ... this can help to trigger concern about signs and symptoms of illness in their pets and prompt early intervention, or a timelier vet visit. The last thing many pets want to do is visit the vet clinic though – unless you are a forgiving labrador! Not all patients are as easy . . .

Melanie was a labrador cross and she wasn't a big fan of the vet clinic.

Robyn was on the phone and sounding flustered. 'Is that Mike?' she stammered.

I recognised the voice. 'Yes, it is. Hi Robyn, how can I help you today?'

'Oh, thank goodness. Look, I've been out at the doctor's and I just got home, and Melanie isn't right.'

'That's no good, what's the problem Robyn?' I asked.

'Well, she's all swollen up like a dairy cow, and she's breathing pretty fast.'

Robyn lived just around the corner, so I asked her to bring Melanie straight down.

It wasn't long before Robyn arrived with Melanie, who had the largest abdomen I had seen for a while and she did indeed look exactly like a dairy cow. A cow has a four chambered stomach and is a foregut fermenter, meaning lots of bacteria ferment the cellulose in grass to digestible fatty acids for the cow to absorb further along the gut. This means they literally have a fermenting vat in their abdomens and normally appear somewhat bloated. But not Melanie. No, this was not normal, and she wasn't coming inside the clinic either!

Robyn had found the cause of the problem on the way out the door and had brought the evidence with her . . . a large twelve kilogram bag of prescription dog food that was unopened before she left home for the doctor's this morning but was only about half full when she returned home! That was a lot of dog food for one dog to eat in such a short time.

Melanie was walking slowly around the car park vomiting dog food as she walked. I could see the similarity between the dog and one of those children's water pistols that occasionally spurted water when the trigger was depressed. The mucous membranes in her mouth were red and congested, which was not

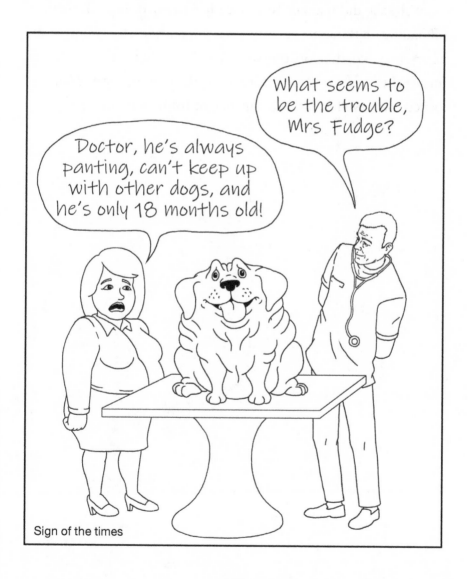

Sign of the times

a surprise. She looked very uncomfortable and was certainly suffering the effects of her overindulgence!

Robyn was not keen on any form of intervention and thought that Melanie would probably offload more of her excess intake on her own. A little concerned with this approach, I advised Robyn to keep Melanie quiet, watch her breathing closely and let me know how she progressed.

Well, she did manage to reduce her payload through further offloading, although she was pretty lethargic for twenty-four hours and did develop the squits, but otherwise she made an uneventful recovery. Not surprisingly, the dog food was securely locked away well above Melanie height from then on!

A wet day

As Napier is a seaside city situated on the east coast of New Zealand's North Island, water sports and all forms of fishing, including deep-sea fishing, are popular pastimes.

Every day when driving out to my farm calls I would pass by the boat saleyard and, being a Piscean, would often stop by to see what was on offer. After a few years of looking, I had a few spare dollars so decided to buy a boat to go fishing in the bay.

After some advice I settled on a Fi-Glass Viscount with an inboard engine. Now, I thought, this should be a bit of fun on the weekends, taking a break and going fishing. I realised later, the best way to enjoy boating is to have a friend with a boat, but now I was that friend with a boat!

We headed out for a trial fishing trip one day, didn't go far out to sea and came back with a small catch. It all seemed to go well.

A fine weekend was coming up, so I phoned my father and brother and they were keen to go out on the boat to do some fishing with me. I had been told that typical fish caught in the bay included gurnard, red cod, kahawai (Australian salmon), sand shark as well as other assorted species. If you fished out a bit further from the shore then you could catch other desirable species like king fish, groper and albacore tuna. These in particular were great eating, so it would be worthwhile on a fine day to venture out a bit further to fish.

As this would be only the second time we had headed out, I thought it best to stick close to the shore, as I wanted to ensure there was no engine trouble, or other unforeseen problems when we were out at sea. We had a fire extinguisher, a marine radio, flares and other safety equipment on board, as well as a small spare outboard motor we could hang over the back in case the main engine failed. Of course, we also had life jackets and a first-aid kit on board. I had purchased some boat fishing rods and the obligatory squid bait and ice to take with us on the day. We were all set.

Although I didn't have the best sea legs, with a fine day and relatively calm seas forecast, I thought all would be well. What better way to start!

The day dawned and we were soon heading off loaded up for our excursion along the shoreline to fish. We made good time planing out over the top of the low waves. Once we had travelled along the shore and out a bit for twenty minutes or so, we stopped, dropped anchor and did some fishing. We baited up the hooks and lowered the lines into the water.

It wasn't long before my brother, Rog, who was fishing at the back of the boat, started getting wet feet. He looked down to see about seven to eight centimetres or so of water on the floor at the back of the boat. I was fishing at the front where there was no water. He called me over, a bit concerned about this.

'Ooo, must be a leak,' I commented as I put the bilge pump on to pump it out.

It was reassuring to hear the whir of the pump, but it wasn't long before the water on the floor of the boat started to deepen even further, despite the whirring of the bilge pump.

A mild degree of panic started to build as we realised that the rate of emptying was slower than the rate of filling, and it was quite some distance to swim to shore!

We hadn't had any bites on our lines anyway, so we hurriedly wound them in and attempted to start the engine to head home. It turned over quite a few times before finally starting, much to our relief.

This didn't look good. I'd just bought the boat and it was leaking. I wasn't feeling very happy, but our immediate concern was to make it to shore before the boat sank! Heading in closer to land first before starting the twenty-minute trip back along the coast to the boat ramp seemed like a good idea.

Luckily, as we picked up speed and gained momentum and starting planing along the water surface, the water inflow stopped. This was just as well because we were literally swimming in water by this point, and my fellow boaties – my brother and father – were busy bucketing water over the back of the boat as we headed back to shore at speed.

Once we got back, we hurriedly backed the boat trailer into the water and winched the leaky boat onto it and drove it back onto dry land.

We breathed a sigh of relief.

It wasn't till we had the boat on the trailer and had driven it out of the water that my brother, Rog, walked around the back of the boat and, glancing down, yelled, 'Mike, did you screw the outlet bung back into the bottom of the boat before you launched it?'

Ask no more questions, the beer was on me that evening!

Third time lucky?

Not surprisingly, any future boating expeditions were preceded by triple checking the bung before departure. In fact, I worried that it would be over-tightened, and I would shred the thread, so we always carried an extra bung.

The upcoming Saturday was expected to be fine again, so I rang my brother.

'Hi, Rog. It looks like good weather this Saturday and I'm not working. Would you like to go fishing?'

'Sounds like a great idea, Mike, I'm keen. Are you going to put the bung in this time though?'

The English locum, John, who was working for me, hadn't been out fishing on the ocean before, so we had a third keen seafarer.

We organised the bait and refreshments, plus some sea-legs tablets in case anyone felt seasick, and set off early on Saturday. We had just recently purchased a long line and attached fifty hooks to it to increase our chances of a catch if our fishing rods were not having any success.

We set off with bung in, motored out to sea and anchored a

fair way out. The anchor went down a good distance, so we knew we were in deep water. We tossed our baited hooks over the side and waited. After a while it wasn't looking too promising, so we pulled the hooks up and decided to do some trolling. This involved motoring along at a slow speed with a line behind the boat, hoping to catch certain fish. Today we had heard that albacore tuna could be caught in this area, and were keen to catch some of these tasty fish. After twenty minutes or so John hooked one and shortly after this my brother Rog hooked another one. They were good-looking fish too, so we were pleased with our catch.

We had no further luck, so after a while we decided to motor in a little closer to the shore and baited up the long-line hooks with squid bait. The idea was for one person – me – to put the boat in gear and motor along slowly while another person – my brother Rog – fed the line carefully over the back of the boat with a sinker attached to the free end to carry the line to the bottom of the sea with the baited hooks strung out behind. After a time on the sea bottom, the line is hauled in over the back of the boat, hopefully with a good catch of fish attached!

We were all set, so off we went slowly. I put the engine in gear by moving the throttle forward and my brother Rog started to feed the line out carefully. The wind had picked up a little and the sea was slightly choppy by now with a bit of a swell, creating slightly rocky conditions on board.

All was going well and Rog was about halfway through guiding the baited hooks over the back of the boat when there was a gust of wind and a rogue wave passed under the boat. Rog lost his balance and while regaining it he momentarily lost hold of the end of the line. He grabbed at it just as it was sliding out the back of the boat and embedded a hook in his finger. Rog yelled at me to put the boat in neutral, but the throttle momentarily stuck in gear and the boat motored forward about ten metres before I could disengage it.

Rog had to jump out the back of the boat as his finger was now attached to the hook and line that was fast disappearing over the back of the boat as we moved forward!

John and I watched with horror as my brother became a large piece of live bait!

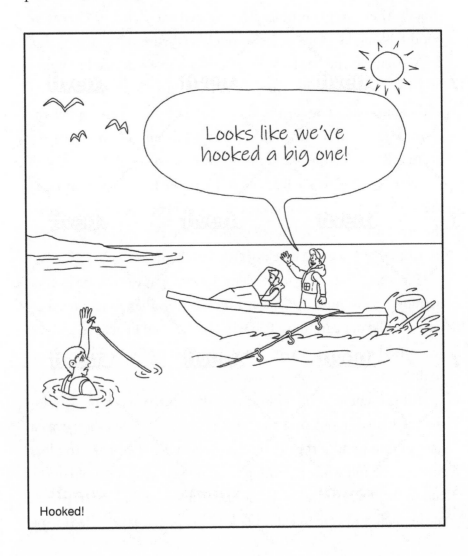

Hooked!

Fortunately, Rog was wearing a life jacket, we were going quite slowly, and the line and sinker were light so there was no major downward pull; Rog was able to float out behind the boat.

We quickly circled around and managed to haul Rog back onto the boat. The poor fellow was soaked, and the fishhook was embedded very firmly in the flesh of his finger!

As anyone who knows anything about fishhooks can attest, they have a nasty barb on them, and they are not designed to be extracted easily. This was an unfortunate turn of events and there was nothing to do but motor back in and head to the emergency department at the local hospital. We cut the line, bandaged the finger loosely and headed back in to shore.

Once ashore, we made a beeline to the hospital. Luckily, it wasn't busy, and the hook was soon removed under local anaesthetic. The emergency doctor made a few wisecracks about why I couldn't remove the hook – 'After all, you must have removed a few from your animal patients surely?' – but funnily enough Rog wasn't so keen on that idea, and I figured the drinks might be on me again tonight!

Rog was a tough cookie, so we decided to head to the local wool store where he worked and lay the line out on the concrete floor to untangle it and cut the bait off the hooks.

We had just finished laying it out when the phone rang. It was Rog's wife, Kerry.

'Hello, Rog, how's the finger love?' Kerry enquired.

'Bit bloody sore,' was the reply. The local anaesthetic was wearing off.

'Well, how about coming home for something to eat? It's all laid out.'

'OK, that sounds great,' Rog replied. Not unexpectedly, we

didn't need much convincing! So we decided to leave the line laid out on the floor and head home for some refreshment and return in an hour or so to finish unbaiting and untangling the long line. Besides, it was the weekend and we would lock the door and be back soon to finish the task.

We had a tasty home-cooked meal with some liquid refreshments, which by this stage was most welcome, and put both our albacore tuna in the fridge for baking the next day.

After the meal, we decided we should head back to the wool store to complete the job. We'd been away for about an hour and a half and as we approached the line it was apparent that World War Three had broken out during our absence. There, to our shock and horror, was a very angry and unhappy black tomcat with a morsel of bait and one of the long-line hooks wedged firmly in the back of his mouth. Horror of horrors! The poor cat. What an unbelievable mess he had created as he had tried in vain to free himself. (It would take us the rest of the day to untangle the line.) I'm sure he had tried all manner of acrobatic contortions to release himself from the hook and line, all to no avail.

What were we to do? John and I had an idea . . .

We headed to the surgery and armed ourselves with an injectable anaesthetic, returned to the wool store and managed to restrain the poor tomcat and anaesthetise him. Once he was asleep, we released the embedded hook and desexed him for good measure. He looked like he was well fed and cared for by some kind soul, but appeared to be a stray, so after an injection of long-acting antibiotic and pain relief we set him free.

I glanced up at Rog, who was looking thoughtful. No doubt he was even happier he'd had his minor surgery at the hospital without extras and not performed by us vets!

Dear Betty

Veterinary science, like many caring professions, is a very satisfying career. We often don't take the time to appreciate, like many people in many different areas of work, and reflect on the positive difference we make to our furry friends and their owners. We need to sit back and take the time to remember this for our health and the benefit of our careers.

But it's not always good news. We are dealing with medical and surgical problems that, by their very nature, don't always respond to treatment, and an important part of our job is end-of-life care and assistance.

Betty had been bringing Benji to see me for about six months with a heart problem. He was a delightful terrier-cross dog who probably was a mixture of Jack Russell, Australian terrier, and a cavalier King Charles spaniel.

Like many hybrid dogs it was hard to tell and often the dog's parents were a mixture of breeds which further complicated the guesstimate. Generally, there is never a shortage of people willing to have a guess. Nowadays there are new breeds of dog created by known crosses and a good example of this is anything with an 'oodle' on the end that has been crossed or bred with a poodle. Labradoodle, cavoodle, schnoodle and retrodoodle are common examples. Most of these make delightful pets and invariably have the health, vigour and relatively non-shedding coat of a poodle hopefully combined with the best features of the other breed.

Benji was about twelve years old and every time he visited the clinic, he was always pleased to see us. His tail would wag non-stop and, like most of our patients, he was very happy to be bribed with treats. Although a treat was not generally required to win favour with Benji.

In the 1980s the mainstay of our medical treatment for congestive heart failure, which unfortunately Benji suffered from, was digoxin and a diuretic (treatment for fluid retention). Digoxin was first isolated in 1930 from the foxglove plant, Digitalis lanata. Among other effects, it helps to increase heart contraction and slow heart rate. It is still used a little in animals nowadays, but with care, as its safety profile and efficacy are not as good as some of the wonderful new heart drugs we have now.

'Good morning, Betty, how are you today?' I enquired with a little trepidation as I knew Benji had been deteriorating lately.

'Hello Mr Small, not so good today I'm afraid. Benji's got me worried.'

'I'm sorry to hear that, Betty. Come on in and we'll have a look at Benji for you.'

I could see that Benji was having a lot of trouble breathing, taking deep breaths in an attempt to get enough oxygen.

I lifted Benji's lip and looked at his gum colour. It was not the normal bright pink of a well-oxygenated body, but a muddy bluish colour, which indicated poor tissue oxygenation. I placed my stethoscope on Benji's chest and heard marked heart murmurs –

Benji was suffering from endocardiosis, degenerate heart valves. I could hear his heartbeat all over the chest, indicating heart enlargement. It wasn't looking too promising for Benji, but Betty did not need me to tell her that; unfortunately it was all too obvious.

'Oh Betty, Benji's mucous membrane colour and his oxygenation level are not good and his breathing is a lot more laboured. I can increase his diuretic pills, but he is already maximised, and his kidney function is not good. Is he eating?'

'No, Mr Small, he's not interested in food now and his belly is swollen. He doesn't want to go for a walk either and his coughing has got worse.'

These were all signs of advanced heart failure. His heart was failing despite all the medication. His quality of life had certainly deteriorated.

'I'm having real difficulty giving him his medication now. I won't have him suffer anymore, Mr Small. I think I need to put him down. Will you come around tomorrow? I would like him to be at home.'

Betty had tears streaming down her face and her usual ruddy complexion was more florid than normal.

This was very upsetting and distressing for Betty, but she knew there was nothing more I could realistically do for Benji. I offered Betty a chair and some tissues and comforted her as best I could.

'I am so sorry Betty. We've tried everything, and it worked for a while but now his heart won't respond anymore, and it's failing. You have been very dedicated, and I know how much you care for Benji. There really is nothing more I can do. Yes, I will come around tomorrow.'

After a while Betty got up and left. It is very sad when there is little more we can do. We are fortunate to have the option of euthanasia when an animal is suffering and there is no hope of improvement.

Poor Betty. She had had a rough time in the last few years. Her husband Des had developed dementia several years earlier and he too was deteriorating, and Betty was still caring for him at home. He frequently wandered off and she had to watch him closely all the time. It was taking a toll on her. The family tried to help but Betty was a very independent and determined woman. As we know it is often the caregiver in these situations who is at risk of ill health due to stress as they focus on their dependent loved one and neglect their own health needs. Betty was not young either.

Making the situation more complicated was the fact that Benji's brother Bruno was also elderly and very devoted to Benji; they had been brought up together and were very close. This is often the way; two siblings are acquired at the same time and spend their life together.

It was a difficult dilemma, but there was no choice. Thankfully, Betty's daughter would be there to provide support to her mum.

The next day came and we headed around to Betty's house. It was a stressful and heart-wrenching time for Betty, but it was good for Benji to be at home in his familiar environment with his brother Bruno.

Betty's daughter Angela comforted her mother and after a while and many treats for Benji we were able to gently euthanise him on his comfortable bed with Betty talking to him.

It went as well as could be expected given the circumstances, and understandably, Betty was very upset. After a while we politely offered our condolences and quietly departed.

This is not the easiest aspect of our job, but one we accept when we graduate as a very important part of it. It is a privilege to be able to offer this service to ease suffering and provide a pain-free and humane end for owners' beloved pets.

Next day the phone went, and my receptionist Anne answered it.

'Mike,' she said, 'you'd better come to the phone. It's Angela, Betty's daughter, she wants to speak to you.'

My heart sank as I rushed to the phone.

'Hello, Angela, it's Mike here,' I said.

'Oh, Mr Small,' she sobbed, 'something terrible has happened. Last night Mum went into the hallway and Bruno was lying there. It looked like he had had a heart attack and just died. Mum was devastated. By the time I got there I found Mum collapsed on the floor, so I called the ambulance, but she died on the way to hospital. The doctor said she'd suffered a stroke.'

I could not believe what I was hearing. How could this happen? It was tragic.

'Angela, I am so sorry, you poor thing. That is shocking news.' I felt absolutely devastated for the family.

Fortunately, this tragic event was never to be repeated in my career, but it is forever imprinted on my memory and serves to illustrate the close bond between animals and their owners and the delicate path that we all tread in this life.

Oh deer

In the 1980s deer farming really took off in various parts of New Zealand and many farms were stocked with wild deer captured after being knocked out with sedative darts from a helicopter. There was a strong demand, and deer commanded high prices. Many farmers hastily converted some, and in a few cases all, of their sheep and cattle land to deer paddocks with the trademark two-metre-high mesh-net fencing. Deer were initially not very tame and required careful handling and mustering. They have improved over the years as they have become more domesticated. Although prices have waxed and waned, a ready market exists for the soft velvet antler considered a health enhancer and aphrodisiac, and for venison. In some Asian countries other parts of the deer are also popular. Many deer farms now pepper the country, with some large blocks farming many thousand head of deer.

Harry Farleigh was a local deer farmer who ran a small block of red deer close to town. He was one of the district's well-known and well-liked characters and he was always playing practical jokes. A young vet was an ideal candidate for him, and he took great delight in cracking jokes about exorbitant veterinary fees and taking the micky, or to put it less politely in farm speak, taking the piss, which wasn't going to be too far from the truth on this particular day.

Harry had a beloved female deer, or hind, who liked to come up and have her chin rubbed and each day he would call her and give her a rub. It was therapy for both of them. She had been hand-reared and had a close bond with Harry. Of course, hand-reared animals can also be more temperamental and Twist was no exception. If she felt like it, she would give you a bite or a push, but fortunately she wasn't prone to kicking out like many of her compatriots! Twist was so called because she was born with a facial deformity which meant she had distorted facial bones and she always looked like she had a wry smile. There was no mistaking Twist.

Harry was to play host to a group of Japanese guests who were travelling around New Zealand as part of a tour and wanted to visit some local farms. Harry being the gregarious fellow he was, had jumped at the opportunity to show them his intensive deer farm and its facilities. He had it all planned. He would first show them his mustering skills before speaking to them in the deer shed. He would then allow them to pat Twist, who was by far the friendliest deer on the property.

The guests arrived and all was going well; Harry was in his element with his whistle in his mouth blowing signals to his two sheepdogs, Yip and Wallow. Every now and again the whistle would drop from his mouth and Harry would yell a not-too-polite command at the top of his voice as the disobedient Yip let the team down.

The group moved up to the yards and we were standing in the loose deer yard with a few of the friendlier deer, and of course

Twist, as Harry launched into the virtues of deer farming and velvet production. Harry was in full flight with the assembled group listening intently when a wave of smiles, then some laughter, broke the audience's silence. It took a while for Harry to realise that he was the source of amusement. At the same time he felt warm liquid well up in his low-cut gumboot. Looking down, there was Yip standing in front of him, leg cocked and midstream, urinating straight into his gumboot!

At this point the incredibly polite gathering erupted into laughter and Yip was given some assistance to get on his way.

Scratch your head

Just as I was about to leave Harry's farm after helping with the talk and enjoying a bit of unexpected humour at his expense, I got a call on the radiotelephone (RT). In the 1980s, there were no mobile phones and if you wanted to communicate from your car to the clinic, the best system was a radiotelephone. It was handy if you were running late or if you had to make another unexpected call while you were in the area, but the reception could be fickle.

It was Anne and she had received a call from Brian Duncan, a local physiotherapist who had a lifestyle block in the Esk Valley, just north of Napier. Brian's Jack Russell terrier, Syd, needed some attention urgently and would I head straight there. This would work well as Brian's property was just over the hill from Harry's farm.

'OK, Anne,' I replied. 'I'm on my way, let him know I'll be there in ten to fifteen minutes.'

It was normally better to have the client bring the dog to the clinic if possible because I might not have the right drugs in the car, but it was on my way back and I could take Syd with me if needed.

131

As I arrived, I was met by Brian and his concerned wife. They seemed quite flustered.

'It's Syd, he's up by the chook house,' Brian said.

I grabbed my kit and we headed up the track to the chook house.

As we approached, I could hear frantic high-pitched barking and panting, and wondered what was going on.

As we got to the chook house, I could see the rear end of a white dog, presumably Syd, frantically diving under the floorboards of the chook house only to emerge backwards soon after. There was a lot of frenzied barking then squealing when he went back under the floorboards again.

I could see there was something under the chook house that he was trying to get at. Undeterred by our presence, he seemed fixated on his mission. It wasn't until I got up close that I could see there was a lot of blood around his head.

Brian finally managed to get hold of Syd and as he turned him around to face me all I could see were two small crazed eyes surrounded by a sea of red bloody scratches! His normally white face, nose and ears were a conglomeration of red-raw bleeding cat scratches, and nothing else. No white hair, everything completely red!

Syd had bailed up a wild cat under the chook house and he wasn't giving up easily! He had been repeatedly diving in and out and pursuing it to the bitter end, but the cat had the better of him. Fortunately, and not too soon for Syd, we had intervened, and the terrified cat ran off. Syd had an unexpected ride to the vet clinic followed by sedation to clean up his badly lacerated face, nose, and ears. He was one sore customer for a while. Totally self-inflicted!

One jab too many

Cyclone Bola, which struck in March 1988, was one of the most damaging storms ever to hit New Zealand and caused widespread flooding and slips on farmland, amongst other things. The worst affected areas were Hawke's Bay and Gisborne–East Cape. In some places more than nine hundred millimetres of rain fell in seventy-two hours. Coastal farms north of Napier, notably steep sheep-grazing country, suffered bad slips and some land was subsequently retired to forestry.

Gus Ramsey had a farm north of Napier on the way to Lake Tutira, an area badly affected by Bola. Gus called me up to blood test his rams for brucellosis. Brucella ovis, the bacteria responsible for the disease, causes an infection of the epididymis (a duct through which sperm passes) of the rams' testicles which can result in infertility. Affected rams need to be culled or they may pass the disease on.

I travelled up there as scheduled on a pleasant day, the job went well and was completed in good time.

'I'll be in touch, Gus, in about a week with the results,' I said as I left the farm.

I had physically examined the rams for any sign of Brucella ovis infection or epididymitis at the same time. They all seemed free of obvious disease and in good health.

About ten days later I rang Gus when the results came in.

'Hi Gus, It's Mike Small here and I have good news. All the rams are negative for Brucella ovis, so we are safe to vaccinate them now against the disease.' Of course, if any of the rams had a positive result they couldn't be vaccinated and would need to be culled. We organised an appointment for me to visit the farm to administer the vaccine.

In those days you could inoculate the rams with two different vaccines on the one day, Brucella ovis and Brucella abortus, which resulted in a good immune response and protection after the one farm visit only, or you could vaccinate them with only Brucella ovis vaccine at the first visit but you then needed a second visit and repeat vaccination four weeks later to produce a good immune response. Of course, farmers and vets preferred the one visit, but the catch was that the Brucella abortus vaccine was a live vaccine and if you accidentally injected yourself you were at risk of developing undulant fever. This is rarely fatal but could result in lifelong recurring intermittent bouts of sickness or fever, amongst other things. There are plenty of stories around of vets who have unfortunately had undulant fever. The safer and wiser vets amongst us would do the two-course shot with Brucella ovis only. In our practice, we were still administering two vaccines on the one day and accepting the risk but making sure we were very careful. Usually. If you did accidentally inject yourself a course of tetracycline antibiotics started within five days or so usually ruled out any chance of developing undulant fever.

It was about two weeks later that I returned to the farm to

134

vaccinate the rams against Brucella ovis with the two different vaccines.

Before we started, I had a word to Gus and mentioned that it was important that we were careful, as I had to administer the live Brucella abortus vaccine.

'Gus, are you happy for me to inject both the vaccines on the one day? If so, we will have to be careful not to self-inject. Or would you prefer I only use the killed vaccine which is safer but will require two farm visits?'

'Na, bugger that. No offence but I ain't paying for two vet visits if I can help it. Go for the two shots and one visit,' Gus retorted.

'OK then, but I have to give the vaccines and we'll need to be careful. Please keep away from the neck and head of the rams as I am injecting them.'

'Righto, no problem,' Gus responded.

We filled the sheep race with some of the rams and worked our way forward in the race injecting each ram in the neck: the Brucella ovis on one side of the neck and the Brucella abortus on the other side of the neck. It didn't take long, but you needed to be careful to make sure you did all the rams and didn't do any twice.

I managed to do one race full with no problems before we let them out and refilled it with the next lot of rams.

Vaccinating the second lot went smoothly until I got about halfway along and struck a few temperamental rams who started rearing up in the air and striking out with their feet. I pushed them down and carried on, but it happened again. This time, just as one of the rams went back down, I went to inject the live Brucella abortus vaccine into the left neck at the same time Gus put his hand on the neck to steady the ram. There was a yelp as the needle shot into Gus's hand. Fortunately, I did not inject the vaccine but of course there would have been some live vaccine on the needle.

'Ah, that was unfortunate timing.' I hadn't expected Gus's hand to be there or that he would attempt to help steady the ram as I injected. He must have seen it rear up and come from behind me to assist.

'Bugger! Are you OK?' I asked.

'Bah, it's nothing. All fine, Doc. Carry on. Just a little prick – nothing I ain't had before.'

I double-checked, and yes, unfortunately it was the live Brucella abortus vaccine, the one that can cause undulant fever.

'Sorry about that, Gus. Wrong place at the wrong time unfortunately.'

'Nah she'll be right, Doc,' he replied.

I carried on and kept thinking about this.

As we finished the job, I turned to the farmer. 'Look Gus, we can't take the risk. You'll need to go to the doctor and get some antibiotics to make sure there's no chance that you develop undulant fever.'

'Nah, I'll be right, mate.'

'No, you may not be, Gus, and we don't want to take the chance. Are you going to town in the next day or two?'

'As a matter of fact, me and the missus are heading in tomorrow, so I'll go to the quack and pick up some antibiotics.'

'Good man, Gus.' I wrote down what had happened and the recommended antibiotic for him to show the doctor.

I headed off after the morning tea and chat with Gus and his wife Heather in the farm kitchen and some light-hearted banter about how Gus would be protected against ovine brucellosis of the testicles now! I told them both about the importance of the preventative antibiotics for Gus and the need to take the full course. They assured me they would see the doctor the very next day.

I went back to the clinic and carried on with the rest of my week, not thinking much more about it.

I was sitting at home four days later when I suddenly recalled the visit to Gus earlier in the week and thought I had better ring to see that he was OK and that the antibiotic course was going well. I picked up the phone and dialled his number.

'Is that Gus? It's Mike here. Are you OK and how is the antibiotic course going?' I asked.

'Oh, g'day Mike, yep she's all good, feel one hundred per cent mate.'

There was a silence before I asked again. 'How's the antibiotic course going?'

'Eh? Nah she's all good, mate.'

'Now, Gus, you did go to the doctor and pick up the antibiotics, didn't you?'

'Nah, she's all good mate.'

Great, I thought, this can't do. I had visions, given my luck, of a feverish farmer in a few days who then developed undulant fever and suffered from a lifelong affliction. There was no choice, I had to head around to his doctor, pick the prescription up, go to the pharmacist to collect it, drive up there and hand the antibiotics to Gus.

So, I got his doctor's name and made a beeline to the very co-operative GP, collected the prescription, drove straight up there, and handed him the tablets.

'You will take the course of antibiotics, starting tonight, won't you, Gus?'

'Yeah, mate, no problem, leave it to me.'

As I left, I wondered whether he would in fact take them because leaving it to Gus hadn't worked the first time. But it was out of my hands now, I'd done all I could.

I never heard any more about it, so I assumed Gus took the antibiotics and that . . . 'She's all good mate.'

A fishy tale

You learn a lot as you go through life but there is something to be said about the naivety or inexperience of youth. Sometimes it can be useful, if not a bit traumatic, to learn a lesson the hard way. Provided no one is hurt! That way you tend never to forget it!

This was true of many of my early veterinary experiences where I just had to get on with solving the problem, learning all the time.

When it comes to a difficult surgical procedure, it very rarely follows the textbook example! If you know the anatomy and have an excellent knowledge of the procedure – and I find it is handy to have the textbook or diagrams in the surgery – you manage to get through it successfully. I soon learnt that what mattered was attitude and perseverance and a belief that you had to solve the dilemma you faced – no one else was going to do it for you. If you adopted this approach, then you would get there. Many a time when a procedure wasn't going as expected or according to plan, the fundamental fact that you had to sort the problem ensured that you did.

This applied especially to gastrointestinal surgery. The same rules applied whether you were dealing with a foreign body obstructing the bowel or removing a growth from the bowel, or something else. Often you had a fair idea of what was going on, but it wasn't until you started operating and got in there, that the full extent of the problem was revealed. Sometimes you had a very strong suspicion that a foreign body was obstructing the bowel, but you couldn't be sure until you saw for yourself.

Nowadays, people walk their dogs along the beach off lead, often distracted by their mobile phones, and often an owner has no idea what their dog has been doing while on the beach. As we know, many of our canine companions are happy to hoover up anything they come across.

Rex was one such dog. He was a large Doberman pinscher and a professional scrounger, and unsurprisingly, he frequently suffered from garbage gastritis. Anything that remotely resembled food was fair game. Whatever Rex had eaten at the beach on this day was not having pleasant effects on him. I am not sure what had distracted Bill, his owner, because mobile phones were still a thing of the future, but he had no idea what Rex had eaten.

Rex stood there in the consulting room with strings of saliva coming from his mouth. He appeared nauseous and was obviously feeling unwell. His belly was very round and swollen but when I tapped it, it sounded hollow and gas-filled. Could he have a gastric torsion I wondered? This is where the stomach rotates on itself and the air that builds up in the twisted stomach cannot escape, or only partially so. The animal rapidly goes into shock and without quick intervention the condition is life-threatening.

'I'm going to need to take an X-ray to check for a twisted stomach, Bill,' I said.

'OK, whatever you need to do, Mike, just do it,' Bill replied.

140

I took the X-ray but could see no signs of a twisted stomach, but there was a lot of dense material and a lot of pocketed gas in the stomach.

Rex's breathing was OK, but, if the gas distention got much worse it wouldn't be long before it pushed on his diaphragm, making it hard for him to breathe, so we needed to act fast.

'I need to give Rex an anaesthetic and see what's going on in that stomach, Bill. I suspect he's eaten something at the beach that he shouldn't have.'

'Yeah, that'd be right,' he replied dryly.

It was a bit surprising that Bill did not keep a closer eye on Rex, given he was aware of his scrounging tendencies. I suppose there is a lot going on at the beach and plenty of distractions, but not being alert when you have an opportunistic pet like Rex is a recipe for disaster!

Bill agreed we should operate, so we made a start.

I put Rex on an intravenous drip and after he was sedated, gave him an anaesthetic.

I passed a stomach tube down his oesophagus and into his stomach but nothing much was released or drawn back up the tube. So, there was no choice but to open Rex up.

Once I had exposed the stomach, I could see it was distended and filled almost the entire abdomen, but it looked a healthy colour and was not twisted.

It was a warm afternoon and very stuffy in the surgery with the hot and steamy sterilising equipment, and the nurse and I surgically gowned up made it worse!

'Well, I'd better open the stomach and see what's going on,' I said.

With that I made an incision in the stomach wall. There was

a loud hissing of gas as the pungent aroma of rotten fish carcass filled the room and we were both nearly overcome with the noxious vapour. This was a case where air-conditioning and face masks, or possibly gas masks, were needed, but unfortunately we had none of those refinements in those early days. Turning my head away and taking a deep breath I asked nurse Debbie to open all the windows and let in some fresh air and to fetch the large stainless-steel bucket from under the table.

Over the next fifteen to twenty minutes we managed to almost fill the twelve-litre bucket with what can only be described as the remnants of a very large fish carcass in the advanced stages of decomposition!

To prevent ourselves from being overwhelmed we took deep breaths and worked quickly before turning away again to exhale and breath in the slightly fresher air away from the open stomach!

Eventually we closed the stomach and flushed the surgical site well, before suturing Rex's abdomen closed.

When he woke up it did not take Rex long to recover. He was soon back to something more like his usual lean self. With that toxic load out of his system there was no way he could fail to feel much better, until next time . . .

A sad affair

Most of the routine farm calls I did were planned, such as the seasonal visits for pregnancy-testing cattle, testing breeding soundness in bulls or rams, removing velvet antler from stags and so on. The other common type of visit was the emergency call-out and this could be anything from a birthing problem through to suturing a horse wound. Occasionally calls were less routine and involved some form of acute distress or freak occurrence.

I have attended several cases of sudden deaths, often in highly valued animals, such as electrocution by lightning strike. The farmer usually has a good idea that this may have been the cause of death as there has generally been a recent electrical storm prompting a health check of stock afterwards. I have seen the electrocution deaths of individual animals, especially if sheltering under or near a tree, and the deaths of groups of animals huddling together under a tree or along a shelter belt where the electricity is conducted along the ground.

But this case was a little different.

The phone rang and I heard, 'Hello, it's Des McIntosh here, I need the vet to come up straight away. I found most of my two-tooth young stud rams dead this morning and I need it investigated. I'd prepared them for sale . . .'

This was one very concerned farmer. He'd gone out to check his stock in the morning and was shocked by what he'd found. How could this be? The weather had been OK, and there'd been no lightning strikes or signs of recent illness to explain the sudden deaths. A vet was needed, at once.

'I'll be up as soon as I can, Des,' I said, concerned.

It was quite a drive, a little over an hour from town on a hilly highway and then along a shingle or dirt road to the farm.

Many of the side roads that ran off the main highway or the main rural roads were unsealed. They had a dirt or clay base with a top coating of shingle, or small stone chips. The county council had maintenance teams who regularly plied the roads with large yellow graders that smoothed the shingle back into a reasonable surface instead of the gouged-out and pot-holed tracks that developed with use. Another problem was that over time, especially when stock trucks used them, the roads developed corrugations, which made for a juddery bone-shaking and teeth-rattling ride, especially at speed. Those of us who used the roads a lot could move along at reasonable speed on the straight stretches, but as they weren't very wide, it paid to slow down around corners because you never knew who might be coming the other way.

I made good time travelling up to Des's farm and when I arrived, we headed straight out to the paddock where the rams had been grazing.

It was a sorry sight and quite distressing to see the perfectly conditioned sheep lying on their sides, dead. Many of them had bloody mouth discharges and diarrhoea, and their limbs were rigid with signs of convulsing prior to death. It certainly looked like some sort of acute poisoning because any of the well-known infectious causes would not have resulted in so many sudden and apparently violent deaths.

I performed post-mortems, recorded the findings, and took samples of various organs and stomach contents for toxicology testing at the laboratory.

It can be difficult to know what poisons to ask the laboratory to test for. You need to be fairly specific and list the tests you require as there is a wide range of possible poisons and testing is often expensive.

Des had some ideas. He had been having a dispute with a neighbour that had turned particularly nasty, and involved threats that had resulted in police involvement.

A common factor with all the two-tooth rams was the drinking water. On farms, this usually took the form of communal drinking troughs. These can vary but often are rectangular or round concrete troughs with a ball-cock valve so they refill when the level goes down. They resemble a small bath and the stock drink freely from the readily accessible water. This made them an ideal vessel for supplements or other more sinister additives!

We wandered over to the main trough. It did look somewhat cloudy and had a faint garlicy smell which I noted might indicate something suspicious. I had taken my poisons book and it did not take long to raise the index of suspicion for possible arsenic poisoning, although this would need laboratory confirmation.

At that time arsenical-based dips to treat sheep and cattle for lice and ticks were still in use, although less so. These dips could still be around in sheep sheds and it was possible that this had been added maliciously to the trough. Unfortunately, it was looking like a strong possibility and Des was convinced this was what had happened. We also took a water sample for testing. I drove away from the farm leaving Des to deal with the awful job of burying his prized two-tooth rams.

Fortunately, malicious poisoning is not common, and I have not had to investigate many cases throughout my career. But in this case the laboratory results came back supporting a diagnosis of arsenic poisoning with a likely toxic concentration in the trough.

This was sad news, but we had some evidence for an insurance claim at least.

I am not sure of the results of the police investigation, but it would not replace Des's prize rams.

Basil who?

I arrived back at the clinic late after this emergency call-out and was running behind time. My colleague was out on farm calls and there was a waiting room full of people, so after a quick clean up, I set about attending to the assembled gathering of clients and pets.

I was aware that I was moving as quickly as I could to make up for lost time, bearing in mind the needs of each patient and my clients, and still trying to provide a thorough and professional service. This was not always easy, but any complex cases, or ones that needed hospitalising, could be admitted and attended to when I had more time, once the initial consultations were finished.

I rushed back into the waiting room to call my next client in when there was an outburst of laughter from one of the clients. Of course, nowadays you'd probably expect to see someone on their smartphone watching a funny video or reading something humorous, but it was the 1980s and no one had cellular phones, let alone smart phones.

Along with the other clients in the waiting room, I turned to see who was laughing.

There in the corner of the room was a middle-aged woman still laughing and staring at me. Hmm, I thought, maybe I have a remnant of the farm call on my clothing or face, or perhaps there's something behind me ...? No, Jessica was looking at me and giggling. After a long moment, she explained.

'I'm so sorry, Mr Small, I couldn't help myself, but you remind me exactly of Basil Fawlty of Fawlty Towers. The way you're running around, darting about and talking at the same time.'

At this point the rest of the waiting room and my receptionist Anne all erupted into a fit of laughter, all at my expense! I had no choice but to join in.

Of course, the part of Basil Fawlty in the TV series Fawlty Towers was played by British actor and comedian John Cleese. Yes, he was a tall lean man with a receding hairline and a trademark moustache who did dart about, although definitely in a less purposeful way! We could all see some similarities, especially now that Jessica had kindly pointed it out! Basil could be described as the incompetent and intolerant manager of the hotel Fawlty Towers, so I was pleased to reassure myself the similarity was visual only.

I made a mental note to slow my pace, convey less urgency and appear calmer when running behind in future. Afterall, we didn't want any more distracting comparisons, now did we!

You never stop learning

Mrs Yarris was a longstanding client who had been a loyal customer of Courtney St George's for many years since he first started practising in Napier in the 1950s. It was now the 1980s and she wasn't the only client who could claim that, but at ninety-three she was certainly one of the oldest.

She had had a succession of pets, initially dogs and then, as she aged, cats. Like many devoted pet owners, her animals were demand fed and smothered with love and affection.

In those days, good commercial diets were not as common as now so many pets were still fed a lot of raw meat. With the emergence of better diets and health care along with the increasing realisation of the importance of our companion animals as family members, average life expectancy seems to have increased. It was my impression when I started in veterinary practice in the early 1980s that an average cat would live for eleven to twelve years or so. Now it's more like fourteen to fifteen years. There were plenty of exceptions to this and like the occasional human who lives to one hundred despite indulging in all sorts of vices, there are a few twenty-one-year-old cats who have only ever been fed gravy meat.

Perhaps they would have lived to twenty-four if they had had a more balanced diet – but that is another question.

House calls were the order of the day for Mrs Yarris as she was largely housebound, but had a few devoted friends who ran errands for her and saw to her needs.

Anne booked an appointment for me to call around to Mrs Yarris's house to check her new cat, which appeared to be a young female.

Gladys, Mrs Yarris's friend, opened the door and greeted me. 'Come in, Mr Small.'

In I went and there was Mrs Yarris as bright as usual standing in the lounge with her walking frame.

'Lovely to see you Mr Small,' she said.

'You too, Mrs Yarris,' I replied.

After the usual chat about the weather and her health Mrs Yarris told me she was a little concerned about her cat. 'I know you're busy, and I hope I'm not wasting your time, Mr Small. I'm normally good at telling what sex a cat is, but Lilly has me a bit stumped.' She had had cats all her life and luckily, despite her age, her eyesight was still pretty good.

'Oh, why's that Mrs Yarris?' I asked.

'Well I can't make sense of it, down there, you know. Maybe my eyesight is failing but I can't work out what's going on. Can you have a look for me please?'

'Of course, Mrs Yarris. I'll have a look now.'

Lilly looked quite big for her age. I glanced down and . . . it was confusing!

Lilly appeared to have ambiguous external genitalia; it looked like a mixture of male and female parts. I could see what looked like a scrotum, but I could not feel any testicles, and there appeared to be a vulva, although this was not normal and could have been almost a penis. I agreed with Mrs Yarris that it was confusing and that her eyesight was indeed still good. She was seeing things exactly as they were.

Either way, it was best to desex Lilly, and as there was nothing to remove externally – no testicles – we would need to operate internally and see what was there! I expected we might find female reproductive organs and that Lilly's external organs were a cross between the two sexes and that she was in fact an intersex or some form of hermaphrodite.

This was all very intriguing to Mrs Yarris and she quipped that even at her age she hadn't seen it all.

'Always best to keep an open mind, Mrs Yarris, there's plenty to learn still!'

'Now, Mr Small, you will help me eat all this food won't you,' she commented as she opened her freezer and started her usual ritual of piling all sorts of frozen meals and assorted goods into a bag for me. 'People are so generous to me and I don't eat very much you know. I just eat a few frozen vegetables and a small piece of fish or an egg for my meal. That keeps me going.'

'No, no, Mrs Yarris, I can't take your food. You've got to keep up your nourishment you know.'

But as usual it fell on deaf ears and I left with Lilly and all sorts of goods in a separate bag. I am not sure what her friends would think if they knew the vet was making off with their home cooking, baking and the supermarket supplies they'd purchased for her, but I had no choice, there was no way I was going to be allowed to leave without them.

The next day I operated on Lilly and she had a normal internal female reproductive tract with uterus and ovaries, but on

151

closer inspection her external genitalia were certainly 'neither one nor tother'. My best guess was that she had an enlarged clitoris along with a penis! Certainly ambiguous. I suspect she was a cat with normal female chromosomes whose external organs developed abnormally due to a surge of male hormones at a critical time in her development. If this were the case, she would in fact be called a 'pseudo' or 'false' hermaphrodite, or feline intersex, which is quite rare (I have seen only two very different cases during my career). Without expensive testing – to no practical end – it was to remain a mystery. Anyhow, as far as Mrs Yarris and Lilly were concerned, the problem was solved.

Dry run

It was a welcome change to drive out through rolling hill country and on to farms, away from the confines of small-animal practice in the city. Companion-animal practice is very rewarding, and it was an area in which I was soon to spend the rest of my working career, but in the early days the panoramic vistas and ever-changing seasons in the countryside were literally a breath of fresh air. I relished getting out and mixing with the farmers and their families. It was certainly an interesting and challenging job, with lots of variety and good old kiwi hospitality.

Part of any successful business involves keeping up to date and adding extra services to your repertoire and it was with that in mind that I was keen to learn more about bull testing. For breeders who sold stud bulls and farmers who wanted to select the most active bulls for mating, an evaluation of bull soundness is important. One of the tests in use at the time, the Blockey test, developed by the Australian Mike Blockey, selected for desirable mating behaviour traits and went hand in hand with other checks such as condition scoring, physical examination and evaluation of semen quality in selecting a breeding bull.

The Blockey test involved setting up several crates in a yard and tethering a cow in each crate and releasing a stud bull into the pen. The number of times it mounted a tethered animal over a short period of time would give you a score of its virility. It may sound inhumane, but the introduced bull being assessed mounts the tethered animal only very briefly before immediately jumping down. The tethered animal is also changed very frequently. This then allows the farmer to select the most active bulls and bulls with any obvious abnormality like penile deviations or hip problems can be culled. This increases the chance of successful matings and higher numbers of pregnancies resulting from the breeding season.

A veterinarian who was an early adopter in New Zealand was Ron Middlemarch. Ron was a well-respected cattle veterinarian who practised in New Zealand's North Island. He was a fount of knowledge on pastoral farming and herd productivity as well as bull breeding and soundness testing. I spent a day with him early on in my veterinary career learning the ropes of bull testing.

There is also a bit of a story about my time spent with Ron. He was a faithful Subaru driver and whilst out with him I made a comment about his current Subaru car and how suitable it must have been for his farm visits. He was very quick to offer me the two following tips, one learnt the hard way.

To clean a Subaru, remove your belongings and open all doors and the boot, turn on the high-pressure hose and hose out the inside of the car, then allow to air dry!

When you buy a new Subaru, stick to the servicing recommendation and make sure you remember to check the oil level!

His car at the time was the second he'd bought recently. He hadn't had his first car very long when one day he was driving on a back-country road and it overheated, then the engine seized. He hadn't topped up the engine oil since he'd purchased it!

Nevertheless, Ron was a great veterinarian who, like many of his colleagues, only too willingly shared his knowledge freely with his fellow veterinarians.

Spring feast

It was a mild late winter or early spring day and I was booked to travel up to Tutira to Neville and Jenny Smith's farm to do some bull testing. A fine day such as this would make it easier to do the job. I had my collapsible crates on a trailer at the back of the clinic, so it was just a matter of connecting the trailer to the car and heading out to the farm. They were heavy but travelled well behind the car and were easy enough to erect once you arrived at the farm.

We set up the crates, strapping them to the sides of the yard, and got started with the testing. All was going well and as usual there was one bull who was a standout, with several others who would be OK to use but were significantly less interested. This was a good result provided nothing happened to the number-one bull between now and the start of the breeding season, but at least there were a couple of backups to share the load!

Once we had finished the testing, cleared the yard, and packed the bull crates on the trailer Neville said, 'Mike, would you like to come down to the farmhouse for lunch? Jenny's expecting you.'

'That sounds like a very nice idea, thanks Neville,' I replied.

So off we went. It was always a treat to be invited in for a cup of tea or lunch as there were some good country cooks out there and usually after several hours of manual work everyone had worked up a good appetite. Besides, it was an important time to catch up and chat to the 'better half', as Neville put it.

As we entered the farm kitchen and exchanged pleasantries with Jenny, there was an aroma of roast meat coming from the oven.

'That does smell good, Jenny,' I commented.

'Well, let's hope so,' she replied as we sat down and started talking about the local news.

It was not long before the contents of the oven were laid on the table for lunch.

Now, being a townie, it wasn't very often I got to taste fresh farm-raised meat or all the unusual or less commonly served delicacies from the farm.

Jenny could see my bewilderment so gave me a run-down on the meal. The oblong structures were 'mountain oysters': the larger ones were calves' testicles and the smaller ones were lambs' testicles. The darker heart-shaped roasted delicacies were lamb and sheep hearts. There were lamb brains, roast lamb kidneys and sections of roast liver as well.

What a line-up! Everyone helped themselves to the tasty offerings with a bit more enthusiasm than the visitor. It was obvious to everyone that this was my first taste of some of these seasonal farm delicacies, but actually, they weren't bad.

Slippery customer

Reverend Jackson sat quietly in the waiting room reading the paper. His much-loved springer spaniel, Roly, now eight years old, sat at his feet. The reverend was a retired local minister, a humble, kindly man with a polite manner. He suffered from crippling arthritis, but never complained, faithfully walking Roly morning and night, despite how difficult it must have been for him.

Roly was not one of my most appreciative patients. A gentle and loving dog at home, his nature changed during his veterinary visits. Like a few of our patients, he did not consider the veterinary clinic one of his favourite places. When the reverend arrived at the clinic, he had first to extract Roly from the car. The dog turned into an immobile lump on the seat and required bribing with treats before he could be removed from the car. This method usually met with only limited success, but eventually, they made it to the waiting room where Roly hid behind a chair, wide-eyed and fearful. A sedative administered at home before the visit made little difference.

'Good morning, Reverend. How's Roly today?' I asked.

'Good morning, Mr Small, well, he's been somewhat out of sorts these last few days, not eating much, and he has a bit of diarrhoea,' the reverend replied.

'That doesn't sound too pleasant for him or you! Come on in and let's have a look at him,' I replied.

To get Roly into the consultation room required a lot of coaxing and eventually he had to be carried in and placed on the examination table.

For some of our patients it is safer for all concerned to place a protective muzzle around their snout. We normally manage to fit one that allows the patient to breath freely, making sure it is not so loose that it can be flicked off with a front paw. Applying a muzzle quickly and correctly the first time is important because it gets progressively harder to fit after each failed attempt. Occasionally a patient won't have a bar of it, and you must then go to plan B, which is normally sedation. Of course, we try to make examinations as stress-free as possible for everyone, especially the patient.

The reverend always insisted on holding Roly while I examined him. He did a good job, and Roly behaved better when his dad was present.

With the muzzle applied we could begin to examine Roly. Our patients can't tell us what's wrong, so it's important to take a good history from the owner and do a thorough examination.

'Reverend, has Roly eaten anything he shouldn't have or been fed anything that could have upset him?' I asked.

'Well, actually, Mr Small, he did grab something on a walk several days ago and I couldn't get it off him before he swallowed it. It looked a little unsavoury.'

This is a common scenario unfortunately; dogs often wolf

down something scavenged on a walk. Some animals will drop what they've picked up, but many will quickly swallow it before the owner can prise it from them. Normally this doesn't cause an upset gut – probably an indication of the robustness of dogs' gastrointestinal tracts.

'Ok, Reverend, thank you.'

On abdominal palpation it was clear Roly was quite tender and gassy. I decided we had better take his temperature, something I knew he would resist!

With the reverend holding on to him I put on a latex glove and lubricated the mercury thermometer. I squeezed out too much lubricant but, oh well, it might make things easier. As I inserted the thermometer into Roly's rectum, he started to perform. He swung his rear end left, right, upwards, downwards, any way he could to try to dislodge the thermometer. In the pandemonium that ensued I managed to lose my grip on the slippery glass tube and with astonishing speed it disappeared into Roly's rectum! It was as if Roly had some sort of retrograde contracture syndrome that sucked in the thermometer. Now what to do? I gently inserted a lubricated gloved finger into the rectum to retrieve the thermometer, which must surely be just inside the anus. I have long fingers, but to my dismay, I could feel no sign of the thermometer. This was a dilemma I had never faced before.

I thought it best to be honest with the reverend as he, of all people, could appreciate how unco-operative the patient was and the reality confronting us.

'Ah, Reverend, it seems, unfortunately, that in the struggle the thermometer has disappeared inside Roly's rectum,' I said apprehensively.

'Oh, oh well, it was a bit of a struggle,' he agreed.

'Not to worry, let's take him outside and I'm sure he'll pass it.'

So out we trotted and for the next ten to fifteen minutes we walked around with Roly, to no avail. He was not going to perform.

'OK, Reverend, do you mind leaving him with me and we'll try again soon. I may have to give him an enema, but don't worry, it will pass, I'm sure.'

Well, logic determined it had to come out, but the idea of a glass mercury thermometer stuck inside his rectum didn't fill me with tranquillity or delight.

'That's no problem, Mr Small, I'll leave him with you. Just give me a call when he's passed it.'

I was thankful that I had such an understanding and trusting client; pity Roly wasn't like his dad!

Despite logic telling me the thermometer hadn't disappeared into thin air, I took an X-ray to see where the slippery customer was sitting. To my horror, the thermometer was sitting very far forward in Roly's descending colon, right up behind his last rib. How could it possibly move so far so quickly?

After a while, Roly still wasn't passing it, so we gave him an enema of warm saline and paraffin. This time he was more co-operative; maybe he realised his predicament! Of course, many animals are better when their owners are not present, so this may have helped as well, although the reverse can also apply, with some patients easier to examine in the reassuring presence of their owners.

After we gave the enema, out we went again with Roly in tow to the front lawn.

This time, it wasn't long before he passed a well-brewed thermometer neatly on the grass.

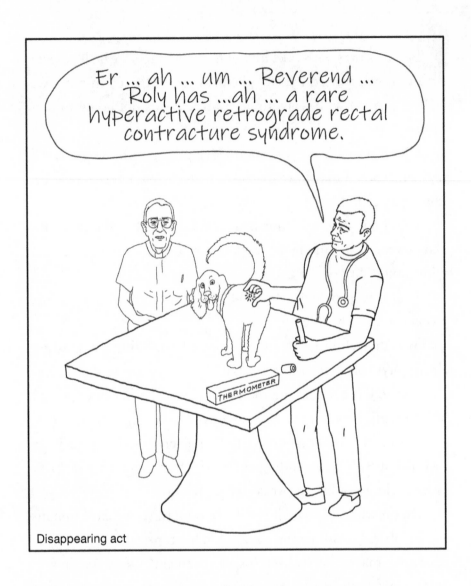

Disappearing act

'Phew, that's a relief,' I said to Debbie.

I called the reverend. 'Hello, Reverend. Good news. Roly has passed the thermometer, and he seems a little better. I'll send him home on a bland diet and some tablets to settle his diarrhoea. I'm sure he'll make a good recovery.'

'Thank you, Mr Small, that is good news. But what about his temperature, did you manage to get that?'

I detected an edge of humour in his voice.

'Yes, yes, it was normal, fortunately,' I replied. I wasn't offering to take it again.

Since that day, I have always carefully lubricated the end of the thermometer only and inserted it only as far as I need to get a reading. You do live and learn. Fortunately, we almost exclusively use digital thermometers now, and although the tip you insert is narrow, the base of the thermometer is much wider and could not possibly go west!

Birthday surprise

Morning and afternoon teas at veterinary clinics can be, from time to time, special. Clients are often very kind and show their appreciation by arriving with unexpected and most welcome gifts of home-baked or store-bought treats. Sometimes it is out of appreciation for a job well done after the patient recovers, or quite commonly, it is at the end of their animal's life after many veterinary visits. Regardless, it is a nice gesture and always much appreciated, but never expected. There are always some great home-bakers amongst your clients and many of us have great memories of individual clients' specialities. Mrs Yarris's friend's bran muffins or Mrs Wright's famous banana cake, for example.

It was my birthday and one of my nurses, Becky, had made a chocolate cake. It looked very good and was sitting in the lunch-room on her grandmother's fine bone-china cake plate and had been nicely iced with candles on it.

Luckily there were no farm calls scheduled and we were all at the clinic; it wasn't busy, so we were all able to sit down for a birthday morning tea together.

Becky had a couple of ageing long-haired dogs, Ruby and

Lucy, and they had come to work today, as usual, for the company and attention. It would be a sad day indeed when the time came to say goodbye to them. Becky was very attached to them and they had formed an important part of each other's lives.

We all sat down with our mugs of tea or coffee and chatted about the day's events so far. Becky was busy lighting the 'few' candles on the cake before bringing it over for me to blow them out. The obligatory 'Happy Birthday' was then sung.

'Very nice, thank you, much appreciated. And thank you, Becky, for making the cake, it looks very good,' I said.

'You've got to make a wish,' they told me, so I did.

Becky proceeded to cut us all generous slabs of the celebratory cake. Why not have a decent piece, it's my birthday after all. It certainly looked moist and delicious, baked last night, and iced this morning before work. No doubt there were a few envious onlookers at home and the dogs today were showing their usual interest.

'Mmm, that tastes good, Becky, thanks for thinking of me and baking the cake,' I said.

As I raised the second piece to my mouth, hanging from the fork and running all the way down to the cake were several long, thick, dark strands! I put the fork down to investigate and pulled out the offending hairs that were well embedded in the cake. No doubt about it, they appeared to be dog hairs! I tried to be discreet, but it was too late, all eyes were on me.

Flushing bright red, Becky said, 'Oh, so sorry, in my haste this morning I dropped the cake on the floor, and it broke into quite a few pieces. I didn't have time to make another cake of course so I moulded it back together before I iced it.'

Mmm, I think the one-second rule for contact time might

have been stretched a bit. With two long-haired shedding dogs, Becky would have been lucky not to have included a few hairs. I appreciated the kindness, and despite the dog hairs, it still tasted good!

It's chocolate time

Talking of chocolate cakes, I recall at university in my first year, when I stayed in a residence hall, there was a first-year student, Rachel, who used to get special packages from her parents. The rest of us occasionally came back with packages, but Rachel's packages were always 'special'. More often than not, inside was a freshly baked cake from her mum. This was stored in the communal refrigerator to keep it from spoiling, but it could be risky with a group of hungry students on hand. The temptation to help yourself was too much to resist for some. By and large it worked out OK for Rachel; not too many noticeable pieces went missing. She was pretty good at offering it around, and I always waited until it was offered, of course!

One weekend, though, it did not go so well for Rachel. On the Friday she had received a package from her parents that contained a very tasty-looking chocolate cake, and this was placed in the refrigerator. A group of male students had gone to the pub that Friday night and returned late. As expected, they had the post-drinking munchies, and had opened the fridge to see what was there. The sight of a freshly baked cake was too much to resist and the whole thing was demolished. They slept well by all accounts.

The next day Rachel and her friends went to the fridge to take the chocolate cake out, but of course it was gone. Surprisingly, there was very little said.

It wasn't too long before another cake, equally tasty-looking, appeared in the fridge.

Unfortunately, it was placed in there before the regular Friday night outing to the pub and sure enough it was almost all gone on Saturday morning after the midnight munchies set in when students returned from the pub. When Rachel came down to the fridge the next morning, she seemed unconcerned that most of the cake had been consumed the night before. In fact, she seemed almost dismissive about it.

It wasn't long before the truth came out, quite literally.

Baked in with the cake was a good dose of senna laxatives that took effect in short order resulting in some gastrointestinally-challenged students walking around groaning for a few days.

Not in the line of duty

We are very fortunate in New Zealand, with a few tragic exceptions, that inappropriate gun use is less common than in some other countries of the world.

However, there are still too many incidents of animals being the recipient of this form of abuse. As veterinarians, most of us over the years have seen far too many slug pellets embedded in patients, mostly in cats. If patients are not presented at the time of the initial injury, the pellets may only be found coincidentally on an X-ray taken for another reason at a later vet visit. The owners are generally unaware their pet has been shot. Often when you find them and question owners, they can recall a time when the cat seemed sore or lethargic for a few days, then recovered without needing a vet visit.

I remember performing one very sad post-mortem on a security dog, Rick.

Rick was a big-bodied German shepherd. In the 1980s there were a lot of the large-framed German shepherd dogs around and if they did not make it as a police dog, they often found a role in security, or as a guard dog. With the right training and discipline,

German shepherds are great working dogs or pets, but in the wrong hands or with the wrong upbringing, they have their share of behavioural issues. With breeders through the early 2000s seemingly selecting for smaller bodied German shepherd dogs, it became harder for those who wanted a bigger dog to obtain them. That seems to be changing now.

Rick unfortunately had the habit of chasing cats, which proved distracting for his owner Bill as well as Rick, and could be a source of embarrassment and frustration at times. And of course it was no less unpleasant for the poor cat being pursued.

However, he was a good working dog and a faithful companion.

Bill rang me one night very distressed. He had been out patrolling and Rick had gone in to investigate a disturbance at a premises and after cornering the intruder had tragically been shot. Could I do a post-mortem and write a report?

This is one of the very sad parts of our job and with a heavy heart I started on the post-mortem.

I could not believe the amount of lead shot in poor Rick's chest. The X-ray I took showed Rick's chest cavity completely peppered with shot. Once I opened Rick's chest the amount of tissue damage was widespread and fortunately death would have been instantaneous.

You could say Rick died doing what he loved and in the line of duty.

It just reminded me that the wrong weapon in the wrong hands is very dangerous indeed. Thank goodness New Zealand and Australia both have strict gun control laws.

Reserve capacity

Most of the patients that we see who have been shot fortunately survive. The unfortunate aspect is the seemingly widespread use of slug guns. They might be fun to use but not funny when used in the wrong manner. Cats seem to be the recipients of more than their fair share of slug-pellet injuries. Often, though, as I've said, slug pellets are a coincidental finding on an X-ray. This is incredible, because there must be pain and discomfort at the time of the original injury, even if the pellet doesn't puncture a vital organ, or strike a particularly painful organ or area. If only our patients could speak, they could tell us what had happened and get some treatment at the time.

Mary was a longstanding and regular client who, like many cat owners, absolutely doted on her fluffy companions. Over the years a succession of moggy cats had the good fortune to cohabit with her. Mary's cats were never left wanting and if she detected the slightest sniffle they were rushed down for a consultation with us at the earliest opportunity. 'An ounce of prevention is worth a pound of cure,' as they say, and this was certainly Mary's philosophy.

Jumbo was a big boy, a grey and white tabby neutered male cat and very friendly. He was the sort of cat everyone loved, who would sidle up to you for a pat, scratch or rub, and who you then had trouble shaking off. Also, and in keeping with his name, he had a big appetite. With some cats you can leave out food and they will just graze on and off all day, masters of self-regulation. Then there are others, like Jumbo, who are not masters of self-regulation and will scoff all the food put out for them at once. Controlled feeding with measured amounts of food is the better way for these fellows. We have all seen and continue to see ten to twelve kilogram cats where the cat has the owners wrapped around their finger, or paw in this case. We try to get the weight of these patients down, but sometimes it is a challenge.

Jumbo was not looking too good on this particular day as Mary presented him to me in the consulting room. He was not his usual friendly self and usually would have leapt out of his cat carrier to come and see me, as he had done at his routine vaccination visit. No, he was definitely quiet for Jumbo. What was obvious was a matted, clumped, blood-stained, raised area of fur over the top of his head. His eyes were dull and bloodshot and his pupil size was a little uneven. He appeared to walk OK but was a little staggery. He looked like he had a big headache.

I took Jumbo's temperature and it was normal. I gave him some pain relief and then we gently clipped away the matted fur on the top of his head. There was a neat round hole underneath.

'What do you think happened, Mary?' I asked.

'Well, I don't really know, Mr Small, I didn't hear any cat fights and he's not usually one to fight. He came in late last night and I noticed the wound on his head. He wouldn't eat his food last night, which is highly unusual for Jumbo.'

'Mmm, normally with a cat fight, where there is a puncture wound, there are two or more bite holes, as the attacker takes a bite, not just the one hole that we have here. Unless of course the second tooth does not penetrate the skin, which is unusual. Often, after a cat fight, I would expect an elevated temperature, too, which Jumbo doesn't have,' I replied.

'So, what do you think it is?' Mary asked.

'Well, Mary, it is such a neat round hole it could be a penetrating injury of some sort. Maybe he has run into something. Or ... is there anyone in the neighbourhood with a slug gun?'

Mary was a bit taken aback by this question and a concerned look came over her face.

'What, you think someone has shot him, you mean?'

'It's a possibility Mary, unfortunately. I think we should admit Jumbo and take X-rays.'

With that, I hospitalised Jumbo, gave him some sedation, and took an X-ray of his head.

There it was for all to see, a slug pellet lodged deep within Jumbo's cranium. What was a shock though, was how deep it appeared to be. On the side view of Jumbo's head, it appeared to be halfway into the depth of his head, which was a fair way into his brain tissue. Remarkably, apart from being a bit depressed and with an obviously sore head, Jumbo didn't seem otherwise to be neurologically compromised, or too abnormal. I could only assume it had missed vital structures on the way through. It must have been fired at close range, though, as it had fractured the frontal or parietal bone on the top of his head on entering. Otherwise, it would have bounced off or become embedded under the skin over the top of the bone. But no, it had travelled well into Jumbo's skull.

I rang Mary.

'Mary, it's Mike here. Yes, there's a slug pellet in Jumbo's head. It appears to have travelled well into his brain tissue but luckily it must have missed vital structures on the way. We will need to operate and remove the pellet, but it could be a bit tricky. I hope it'll be easy to find otherwise we could be in a bit of trouble, but I'm hopeful it won't be too difficult to remove.' I did have my doubts though.

'Oh, that sounds ghastly!' A very worried Mary came down to see Jumbo before the surgery just in case things did not go well.

We anaesthetised Jumbo, clipped the fur, and gently prepared the area for surgery. It was a small entry hole which I had to enlarge slightly with a mini craniotomy to allow me to explore a little further. Once we had gently flushed the area with saline and removed the fur that had been carried in by the pellet I was able to probe down with a pair of thin-nosed forceps. It seemed that the forceps just kept sinking further and further into Jumbo's brain tissue and I was getting a little uneasy, but there was no resistance as I gently inserted them. After carefully directing and probing, the tip of the forceps settled on something hard and metallic that was quite different to the surrounding tissue. Luckily, I was able to open the forceps and grab the offending slug pellet and withdraw it carefully. This was a hallelujah moment; we were so pleased. After flushing the cavity thoroughly with saline, packing it slightly and suturing the skin over the defect, the surgery was finished and Jumbo made a good recovery. He didn't appear mentally compromised at all and was soon back to his usual tricks . . . quite amazing! Jumbo wasn't the only one who was mind-blown!

Late for school

Shingle roads were the rule, rather than the exception, once you turned your car off the main highways that led to and from Napier. Often, when you first turned off, a kilometre or two of road would be sealed, then suddenly it changed into the classic rural shingle or dirt road. Mostly, these were graded at regular intervals by the county council, but they soon became corrugated again. Nevertheless, you could travel at reasonable speed on the straight stretches of these roads. Often in summer the telltale clouds of dust hanging in the air along the road ahead would tell you that there was a vehicle in front of you and you knew to stay well back. Even if you put your car's ventilation system on recycle and shut the windows the fine cloud of dust still sneaked in to the car's interior. On a hot summer's day air-conditioning is very handy, and of course all cars have it nowadays, but in those days, summer could be a bit unpleasant without it. Often, after you hit the shingle road, it wasn't long before someone appeared in front of you, in no rush to get home. There was, of course, a high chance that you knew the person driving in front of you, so it paid to keep a respectful distance behind and to drive considerately.

Trouble was you were always rushing and they normally were not.

A large proportion of the roads had some sharp or blind bends on them. Most of the roads were not much wider than single lane, or at most one and a half car widths wide! As you can imagine this made for interesting driving, especially if you met someone coming the other way on a blind corner. Keeping your speed down and keeping left were pretty much the gold standard rules.

I was heading out to do some pregnancy-testing on Richie Blake's farm directly west of Napier. The road out there was notoriously long and winding with hilly undulations. Fortunately, the main road, although just two lanes, was sealed, so you could make good time if you kept left and paid very close attention to your driving. After turning off the main road there was a good length of sealed road before you drove onto the inevitable shingle road.

I had been held up at the clinic with an urgent call and was running late, as happened quite frequently. The desire to make up time on the road needs to be resisted, nevertheless, I still tended to push it a bit.

Today was no exception. I had made good time on the sealed roads and turned onto the shingle road into Glendale farm, which was narrow, relatively flat, but very winding with lots of blind corners. It was a fine fresh day, ideal for pregnancy-testing. Normally at this hour the road was deserted, but you could not rely on it. There were a series of dog-leg bends to the left around a small hill where the road was only single lane.

As I rounded the tighter of the left-hand bends, keeping left, a large red and cream Bedford school bus suddenly appeared right in front of me, coming straight at me. There was literally nowhere to go so I slammed on the brakes. This sent the car sliding to the right and I braced for the impact. It was a low-speed collision but modern Japanese car versus 'solid as a brick sh**house' Bedford school bus meant I was the loser. School buses are not the best vehicles to hit for another very good reason . . . they generally contain unrestrained school children as well as the driver. And what's more, the school children of the small rural community and probably of the farmer I was just about to visit!

I got out of the car and the driver stepped down from the bus to survey the damage. As we had collided at low speed I had made very little impact on the bus or its occupants. Fortunately, all the passengers were fine. What was interesting was that there was absolutely no dent or any damage visible on the bus, but the right-hand front of my car was pushed in! Luckily, it was still just drivable, and with a few running repairs and some profuse apologies, it was not long before I was on my way.

When I got to the farm Richie and his workers knew all about it. Presumably, the bus had a radiotelephone and the news of the day had already been broadcast around the local community. It was certainly a lesson to keep speed down on these rural roads because local news travelled at great speed!

Now I am older, I think back on those early days in practice, and the misplaced feeling of the indestructibility of youth, and realise how much those notions needed tempering. It makes me grimace now to think about it.

It wasn't the only time the farm-call vehicle required some bodywork! Wandering stock on rural roads can be a hazard for anyone, including the animal. Normally, if farmers graze stock along the roadside they place signs, or a shepherd is watching and warns approaching vehicles. Stock do manage to escape occasionally through damaged fencing or gates, especially after storms or if a gate is left open. The larger the animal the greater the risk for the driver and animal.

It was not long after that incident that I was travelling along the same main road west of Napier to a farm call. I came around a corner, over the brow of a hill and right there in the middle of my lane was a large ewe. There was no time to avoid a collision and the resultant impact did not bode well for the sheep or my vehicle. There was a large dent in the front left of the car and the radiator was ruptured. I was lucky, though, as there are plenty of stories of cows or horses on roads and the outcome for driver and animal is not so good.

One of my colleagues, John, told a humorous story of a solo incident in graphic detail. As usual he was running late and was doing the wrong thing by trying to make up time on a country road, and of course it was a shingle road. There was a straight stretch of road along the top of a small ridge of low hills and that day he was, as usual, going a bit faster along the straight stretches then slowing down just in time for the corners. Unfortunately, this day he left his braking too late and went flying off the end of the road, becoming airborne over the top of the farm fence and landing on all four wheels in the paddock below. When he came to a stop, he was sitting neatly in the middle of the farm paddock surrounded by curious stock. Luckily, no one was hurt but he had to suffer the indignity of being towed out by the farm tractor and spent some time reorganising the contents of his car, as his veterinary kit had been tossed all around the vehicle.

Another commonly encountered hazard is the county council tractor that has a mower attached at the back and plies country roads mowing the berm or grassy shoulder of the road. These drivers must be very skilled as they are constantly dodging ditches and undulations, not to mention fixed objects like trees and rocks. They normally place signs warning drivers that they are mowing grass ahead, so you are warned. Occasionally there is no sign, or it has blown over, or you just don't see it. Fortunately, I have not run into the back of a council mower but had a near miss one day when I came around a corner and there it was, the council mower taking up two-thirds of the lane I was driving in. Luckily, I was able to swerve into the oncoming lane and drive around the mower as there were no vehicles coming towards me. I dare say these tireless drivers have some hairy stories to tell. Fortunately, most drivers on rural roads are used to the conditions and remain alert and drive to the conditions, including (most) vets running late!

Tying times

———

Dr Google is part of our everyday life now. It provides a great source of information for all of us. Sometimes, though, it needs to be read with caution and interpreted with care. Occasionally clients will ring having already googled their pet's symptoms and arrived at a diagnosis. Occasionally, they have been administering some home treatment, or they know what's wrong with their pet and just want some treatment dispensed. Often, though, the diagnosis is wrong, or it may be one of many things and needs a veterinary visit and appropriate diagnostic tests. It is not difficult to convince these clients to come for a visit as by this stage there is normally a good reason for the phone call – Fluffy is not getting better! Fortunately, it is more common for clients to ring and book an appointment and come in with ideas about what is wrong, thanks to Dr Google. We all do this and it's not a bad thing; it always helps to have an owner who has some knowledge of the possibilities and some understanding of potential diagnoses.

Occasionally, we get a client who appears to have obtained their veterinary degree on-line and knows what the problem is, and the treatment required . . . We all like to have a punt at what's wrong but often even the most brilliant diagnostician requires diagnostic tests to confirm or deny suspicions! A common one here would be a pet who is drinking more than normal. This could be anything from kidney or liver disease or urinary tract infections to hormonal imbalances or diabetes, to name a few. As vets we often don't know what's wrong until diagnostic tests are performed.

Before Dr Google, we used to get more enquiries asking us to explain symptoms or occurrences that puzzled our clients. One of these came from Mr Ramsay.

'Mr Small, we've got a problem. We meant to get Kendra spayed but she came into heat before we could get her booked in with you. Now the neighbour's dog has just slipped into our yard and mated with her and they are out there stuck together. We can't separate them Mr Small. Something's wrong and we don't know what to do. We've thrown a few buckets of cold water over them, but it hasn't helped, and now they are facing different directions, but still stuck together.'

Nowadays this sort of phone call is very uncommon. Maybe it is because everyone is more informed, or maybe it is because people rush inside and google 'dog mating' and learn that this phenomenon of 'tying' is normal in dogs.

Interestingly, the dog's penis has a glans penis near the base, which at the time of mating swells up and results in a period during which the dogs are tied together. This is normal, and if left alone, after fifteen minutes or so they will untie and can go their separate ways.

'That's OK, Mr Ramsay, you don't need to worry, that is totally normal. Often dogs are tied together for a period of time after mating. Just leave them alone and they will part in their own good time.' There was an audible sigh of relief on the other end of the phone.

The next question that often follows is 'How do we avoid Kendra falling pregnant?' If this is not asked or discussed at the time of the emergency phone call, it's often not long before the phone rings again with this next question!

Fortunately, there are drugs – so called 'mismating injections' – that can be injected at certain times after mating. Formerly oestrogen injections on day three, five and seven after mating were given, but they were not always successful at preventing an unwanted pregnancy. More importantly, the incidence of subsequent adverse complications was unacceptable so they have been discontinued. Now, a much safer drug is available, not surprisingly at much greater cost. This is generally given several weeks (usually at least three to four) from the time of mating.

Many clients, just like the Ramsays, were going to get their dogs spayed anyway, but the bitch jumped the gun, so to speak. Many opt to wait several weeks until their dog has finished their heat, then spay them in the early stages of pregnancy. If the owner doesn't wish to spay them when they are pregnant but wants to let the bitch have a litter of puppies, then a clinical examination, ultrasound or blood test, or a combination of these at three to four weeks after mating can be used to confirm or rule out a pregnancy. Once again, even after the incident, timing is of the essence.

It happens to us all

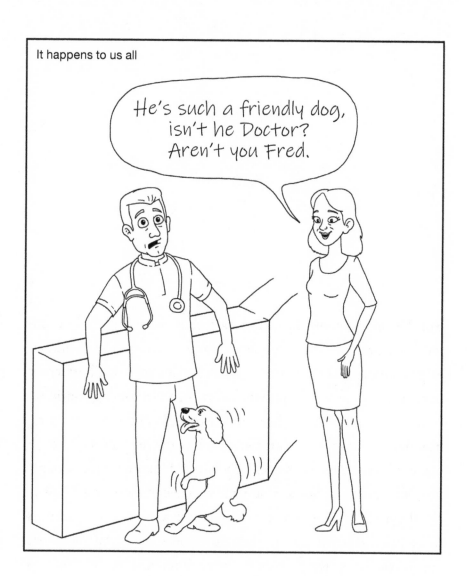

Farm kill

Ron Tilson had come into the clinic to buy sheep drench. Drench-ing is the practice of using a drench gun to give a dose of anthel-mintic (anti-parasitic worm) drench by mouth to kill internal parasites such as intestinal worms. It is carried out regularly on farms and is particularly helpful for young lambs and calves who have less resistance and are more vulnerable to worms. Drench companies compete with each other and often offer big discounts or bonus product, but at that time it was common to give away small appliances like toasters, jugs, sandwich-makers, crockpots or even saucepan or cutlery sets. Appliances were relatively more expensive then so the promotions often lured farmers in. Ron was no exception and his wife Gabby had sent him off to town with firm instructions to call by and collect the deal.

'Morning Ron,' I said.

'G'day, Mike,' he replied.

We organised the drench and Ron expressed some concern about his calves and young steers.

'They aren't thriving, I think we need to do some tests. I've been drenching them regularly, so it's not worms.'

'OK, Ron, how about next week for a farm visit?'

We settled on a date and time.

When the day came I travelled up to the farm. It was always interesting and sometimes gently amusing to visit Ron's farm as there was one definite pecking order on the farm and another inside the farmhouse. There was a quite clear definition of roles between Ron and his wife Gabby with one or other always trying to encroach on the other's domain. This resulted in some interesting exchanges between the two of them.

Ron had a booming authoritative voice and a stare that he fixed on you as he barked commands. It was all very serious. In saying that, if things became too difficult or weren't going to plan it led to either a frustrated outburst of yelling or an eruption of laughter and you were never quite sure which way it would go. Gabby seemed to take delight in baiting Ron when they were outside the house, but the reverse applied inside the house; then it was Ron's turn. It was advisable to stay out of the line of fire and keep quiet!

I arrived on time as the stock were being rounded up in the paddock to bring into the yard. 'Get in behind' is a common command for sheepdogs and Ron had free use of this today, as his disobedient sheepdogs were, as usual, a bit wayward. Dog training wasn't his forte.

The stock certainly looked small with rough, light-coloured coats and there were signs of ill thrift – when stock do not grow at the usual rate. Some of them also had diarrhoea. This could be caused by several things, but we certainly needed to check for worm resistance and mineral deficiencies amongst other things. I set about examining them and collecting faecal and blood samples. It was going well, and Gabby was helping to fill up the race with stock. According to Ron, Gabby wasn't doing it correctly. He was barking commands and staring her out. I suspect it was a bit of a game between them, but to an outsider it was best to keep your head down. I was always worried that if I intervened, I might get an earful!

In saying all this Ron had a good heart and once the job was done and he could relax he liked to have a good chat about the usual farm and off-farm topics.

The sampling went well and with the job done, we went into the farmhouse. This was Gabby's domain and the commands now came from her. Dirty boots and clothes had to come off, hands had to be washed outside by the door and Ron was to sit down and let her provide the refreshments. If he tried to interfere or help too much he was told to be quiet and leave it to her. It all seemed to work well and there was a system, even if each of them tried to test the boundaries.

As we were enjoying morning tea, including some of Gabby's famous savoury cheese scones, Ron asked, 'How would you like some fresh turkeys to take home, Mike?'

I hadn't been offered anything like this before and as he spoke, I had visions of the Christmas turkey, cranberry sauce and gravy on the table.

'That's very generous of you, Ron. That would be nice, thank you.'

'All organised then, we'll get you some on the way out.'

Now I had visions of some freshly killed prepared or frozen turkeys.

We finished our tea and headed outside.

'Right, let's head down to the paddock and we'll get you those turkeys,' Ron remarked.

OK, I thought, the paddock?

So off we went.

Ron rounded up the turkeys and within a short space of time had killed four of them for me. I was a little taken aback and embarrassed at my naivety, although Ron did not realise this as I wasn't showing my surprise.

I had a few containers or buckets in my car, a station wagon. Ron had removed the heads and necks and deposited them upside down in my buckets. I left for town with four turkeys, neck down in buckets, with their feet, rear ends and feathers sticking upwards in the air. To those with a slightly warped sense of humour this did look a bit comical and I have images in my mind of the feathers and turkeys swaying around from side to side in the back of my car on the winding road back to town.

Once I got home and had time, I recruited some help and we set about plucking and preparing the turkeys. This took some time as they were not small and there were a lot of feathers. We froze three of them and decided to cook one for dinner.

The experienced among us would by now have an inkling of what was to come.

After following the roasting instructions for a turkey, the dinner was laid on the table. It looked interesting. Certainly, the colour of the turkey was somewhat darker than the Christmas turkey and the aroma was stronger as well. As we began to slice the turkey the knife did not go through as expected either. This was starting to look a bit ominous.

As we attempted to cut up the turkey on our plates we had a premonition of what was to come. Steak knives were fetched and even then the meat resisted our efforts – it was as tough as old leather boots!

What's more, the flavour was pretty strong when we did manage to taste it.

Unfortunately, once again, even the dog wouldn't eat them.

I learned much later that freshly killed turkeys have to age for a day or two to avoid toughness, and that there's an oil gland near the tail that must be removed to avoid it spoiling the flavour. Tot that one up to experience.

Summit time

Calving and lambing season in the early spring is a very busy time on a farm with multiple newborns arriving in quick succession. Things don't always go smoothly. It can be a time of changeable weather and in some parts of New Zealand, especially the South Island, but also the high country around Napier, snowfalls can mean freezing conditions or difficulty in accessing stock. Farmers can be out checking stock for birthing difficulties any time of the day and night and rescuing newborns separated or abandoned by their mothers for some reason or other.

On one such night the phone rang at ten o'clock.

'It's Paul Jackson here, is that Mike?'

'Hi Paul, yes it is, how can I help you?'

I knew it probably was not going to be anything straight-forward at that hour of the night. Paul was not inclined to phone unless he had to, nor was anyone else for that matter. Experienced farmers are pretty good at handling the uncomplicated problems associated with birth themselves, so I knew Paul had probably tried to resolve the problem before picking up the phone and calling the vet.

'Good, I thought it was. Listen, Small, one of my prize cows is having calving problems. Can you come up now? I've got her in the yards.'

I had a lot on the next day at the clinic and Paul was a good hour and ten minute drive from Napier on a winding hilly road. What is more, I would have to drive to the clinic first and pick up some gear. But that is the reality of rural veterinary practice and spring could often be a busy time of year. Veterinary practices that service a lot of dairy farms are very busy in springtime with calving and metabolic problems like milk fever (low blood calcium), hypomagnesaemia (tetany or grass staggers) and ketosis (when energy demands – milk – exceed energy intake – feed). Fortunately, there were not many dairy farms in the practice, but valuable beef breeding cows still resulted in a few emergency call-outs. It was not always during the day, either, but that was the nature of the job and farming.

It was not the best weather that night. A bitterly cold wind was blowing with scattered rain showers and it was not going to be any better on the top of the ridge where Paul's cattle yards were located! I put on an extra layer of clothing in anticipation of this and headed to the clinic to load up the car with what I thought I would need. You had to think clearly and anticipate all eventualities because it was a long way back to town to collect a forgotten essential!

I headed up to the farm, making good time because at this hour there was little, if any, traffic on the road. As I drove, I noticed the weather wasn't improving; in fact it was deteriorating! I hoped that it would be an easy and quick job.

When I arrived, I got the usual welcome and witticisms.

'Hello, Small, I suppose you were just about to head to bed were you when I rang?'

'Well, as a matter of fact I was, Paul, but that's what I'm here for.'

'I hope you're not going to add an extra zero to the bill then, eh?'

This was said with a wry smile, but of course there was the usual general concern about the veterinary bill!

'Any extra I'll send to the weather gods, eh Paul? They're not on side with us tonight are they?' I said.

That got a chuckle.

Paul's shepherd and assistant Andy had dragged himself out of his single man's quarters looking a bit the worse for wear. There was a local pub down the road that was probably his regular watering hole. After work there wouldn't be much to do, and it could be a lonely existence for a single shepherd on remote country stations in those days with little social media, so the local pub provided a point of contact and social interaction. The publicans were often larger-than-life characters and they more often than not enjoyed a few beers as well. Pubs were scattered all over the countryside then, but there are less of them nowadays with better roads, declining profit margins and dropping rural population. Andy always had a roll-your-own hanging out of the side of his mouth and his nicotine-stained fingers and chesty cough were testament to his long-time habit. Andy, like his boss, enjoyed a good laugh and it was often at the expense of the visitor, or vet in this case.

We walked to the yards and I got ready with my rectal gloves and calving gown over the top of my extra layer of clothing. There certainly was a biting wind in the yards, and I hoped the problem could be resolved quickly.

As we approached the cow in the race another gust of wind and a squally shower added a sense of urgency.

My heart sank as I noticed a discoloured discharge coming from her vulva. Ruth, as she was named, was standing, and seemed reasonably strong and otherwise in good condition, which were promising signs.

'How long has she been calving do you know, Paul?' I asked.

'We just spotted her today,' was the reply.

This being the case she was obviously a few days overdue and it was likely the calf was not alive.

'She's one of me good breeding cows,' Paul added, 'and I don't want to lose her.'

'Yes, I understand.'

I lubricated my gloved hand and arm and performed an examination.

It did not feel hopeful and unfortunately the calf was dead and starting to swell. There was not anything to do but to remove the calf from the cow to save her from likely toxaemia and death.

'I'm sorry Paul, but the calf is dead, and we will need to do a foetotomy and remove it to save her.'

'I thought as much. Well, you'd better get on with it then, Small, hadn't you,' Paul said, a wry smile on his face.

Now a foetotomy is not the most pleasant of things for all concerned as it involves sectioning the dead calf with a foetotome which is essentially a looped piece of 'giggly wire' that extends from a protective hollow pipe. This is inserted into the cow and used to gradually section the calf and remove it as you do so. If the dead calf is left inside the cow, she will most likely not survive.

It proved to be a difficult task as there was not a lot of spare room to manoeuvre. The next hour or so was peppered with repositionings, sweating (despite the conditions), and a barrage of

'Come on, Small, jeepers, we haven't got all night.' The smiles started to fade as time went on and halfway through Ruth decided to lie down, which did not help. The yards were muddy as well which added a further twist to the night's activities.

After what seemed to be a painfully long time during which a pair of earmuffs would have been handy to deflect the barrage of jibes, the job was done. Ruth received some antibiotic treatment amongst other things, and she was as relieved as we were the process was over.

'Well, Small, I don't know what took you so long. She'd better survive.' This was delivered with the slightest of wry smiles, but the underlying meaning was pretty clear. 'I don't want to get a big vet bill for a dead cow; in fact, I don't want either.'

'Well, Paul, it's up to her now. Keep her out of the elements and give her some supplementary feed and the medicine I'm leaving with you and give me a ring tomorrow and let me know how things are. We've done all we can for now.' It was a pity we'd been too late to save the calf, but at least Ruth seemed OK.

Thankfully, Andy arrived with a bucket of warm water, soap and a towel plus a thermos of hot chocolate. That was a welcome treat after a difficult job. After a hurried clean up and drink, we all quickly retreated to warmer environments. It was not until I arrived back in town with the heater in the car on full that I started to warm up.

I rang Paul the next day and fortunately the news was good, and Ruth continued to make a good recovery in the days ahead.

Paul paid the bill, no zero added!

Insult to injury

Zoonoses are infectious diseases that are transmissible from animals to humans. In New Zealand there are not as many zoonoses, nor in general are they as life-threatening, as zoonoses in a lot of overseas countries. Rabies is not present in New Zealand and long may it stay that way as this is a fatal disease. Campylobacter, a gut pathogen causing gastroenteritis, and salmonella, can be caught from several animals, including cows, but normal hygiene precautions should prevent this in most cases.

On a cold, cloudy autumn day I headed up the Napier–Taupo road to Gary Saker's farm. Like many farms, it was several kilometres off the main highway and down a shingle road. Luckily, it only served two farms, so I was not very likely to meet vehicles coming the other way, which was just as well on such a narrow and winding road. Yes, there was a school bus that plied the road, so an abundance of caution was necessary. On arrival there were the usual group of barking sheepdogs that escorted me in, and when I came to a stop a fair amount of investigation of the interesting smells that the vet brings in. The obligatory sprinkling of the car tyres followed, leaving their telltale trademarks.

Next came the usual exchange of greetings with the farmer. There were not too many cows today, but they were 'a bit wound up' for some reason. If the day were windy it could have affected the stock, but I suspected it was the frenzied herding of the cows into the yard and the sense of urgency that had them agitated. A gentle approach always helps, bringing the stock near the yards the day before, then herding them in quietly the next morning, but of course this is not always possible. Anyway, they were not looking too settled and I was probably in for a jostling.

'How's things, Gary?' I asked.

'Not bad, Mike. Could do with a bit more feed going into winter,' he replied.

It had been a dry summer and there had not been much rain so far this autumn, which was not unusual but meant less feed reserves and more supplementary feed needed.

As the pregnancy-testing season goes on and as the years go by the chance of either an acute injury or an RSI (repetitive strain injury) from pregnancy-testing increases. There are much more dangerous jobs out there but on a day like today with unsettled cows the risk of injury is heightened. It was not long before a particularly feisty cow was penned, and my arm got a good wrenching from the rear-end dance she was performing. The brisk repetitive left to right and right to left movements wrenched my elbow and caused triceps tendonitis.

'I say, Gary, the cows are a bit frisky today, you reckon?'

'Yeah, I reckon it's the weather, Doc.'

Well I was not sure if it was the weather or the yarding technique, but maybe it was a bit of both.

It was not long before my left arm got another good wrench and it took a few minutes to settle.

I had only tested another four to five cows when, as I walked in behind a cow, she lashed out with her back leg and kicked me on the front of my thigh with maximum force. I recoiled in pain and had to step out and lift my leg off the ground. After several minutes I returned to finish the last few before retreating to the farmhouse where a bag of frozen peas served as an icepack for a while.

Gary's Scottish upbringing taught him that the best thing for pain was a good shot of whisky, so out came the kitchen tumblers and a generous glass full of straight whisky was handed over, along with shortbread and a strong cup of coffee. That seemed to hit the spot and dull the pain. I was in no state to say no – I needed something to ease the pain in my throbbing thigh muscles.

After I arrived back in town it was more icepacks and elevation. Over the coming weeks I needed to see our local physiotherapist to get the leg moving again and disperse the haematoma that had formed in the muscle. The pain at night was unpleasant for several weeks, likely due to pressure from bleeding into the muscle, so I developed great sympathy for my animal patients who suffer the same affliction.

It was not to be my only haematoma from pregnancy-testing, but I soon learnt to be careful when walking behind even a seemingly calm animal.

To add insult to injury it was about a week later that I came down with campylobacter gastroenteritis, which was most unpleasant, as anyone who has had it can attest, and this resulted in a good week off work. It was the only time I ever had it, and I lost three kilograms before I recovered. I presume that my hand hygiene had slipped up somewhere along the line after pregnancy-testing so there were two lessons to be learnt the hard way in a very short space of time.

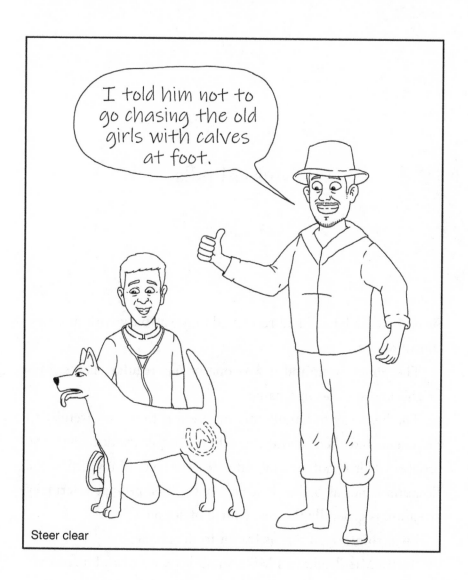

Steer clear

Musical pills

Several weeks later, I had recovered and was busy with morning consultations.

The phone went and it was one of our regular clients, Mrs Bright, and she was in a panic.

The best way to handle this situation is to listen carefully to the client and then advise them how to quickly deal with the problem. If it is not serious, offer reassurance. Many times, the situation is not as bad as it seems, but if it is, prompt veterinary attention is generally the best course of action.

I was thinking of this as I went to the phone.

'Hello Mrs Bright, it's Mike Small here, how can I help you?'

'Mr Small, a terrible thing has happened.'

There was silence and panicked breathing on the end of the phone.

'It's OK, Mrs Bright, I'm here to help you, what is the problem?'

'Well, I got up a bit late this morning and went out to the kitchen, got my pills out and took them. Then I got Gyp's tablets out and gave them to him. It was not till I was having breakfast that I looked over to where the pills were and saw my pill bottle sitting on the bench where I had dosed Gyp. I realised that I must have given Gyp my tablets and I took Gyp's pills! What am I to do Mr Small? This is terrible. I feel so stupid and I'm very worried ...'

Now Gyp was a west highland white terrier who weighed about ten kilograms. Mrs Smart was an elderly, rotund woman probably seven to eight times Gyp's weight, so I was not so worried about the fact that she had taken Gyp's tablets, not that I was a human doctor. I knew that Gyp's tablets were prednisone, five milligrams, which for a human being was unlikely to have any major ill effects, unless she had taken a few of them, but even then, the effects probably were not going to be major.

'How many of Gyp's pills did you take, Mrs Bright?'

'Only one, Mr Small.'

'That's probably OK, then – it's a pretty safe tablet and a low dose for you. You should be fine, but please ring your doctor to check.'

'Thank you, Mr Small.'

'Now tell me what tablets you take, Mrs Bright, and how many you gave to Gyp please.'

'It's my thyroid pills, Mr Small, one tablet.'

This could mean several things – did Mrs Bright have an overactive or underactive thyroid? I assumed they were likely to be thyroid replacement tablets as this is a common medication for humans, and animals.

'Mrs Bright, what is the name of the tablets and the strength?' I asked.

'It says here, thyroxine fifty mcg.'

What a relief.

It seems that the human dose of thyroxine is, in general, much lower than the dose we use for thyroid hormone replacement in animals. Humans seem to be on maybe one to two micrograms per kilogram, but our animals are commonly on a ten to twenty micrograms per kilogram dose. In other words, they normally receive ten times the dose per kilogram of bodyweight. This was a stroke of luck I thought.

'You can relax, Mrs Bright, that dose of thyroid hormone supplement for Gyp is unlikely to cause a problem. It might make him a bit agitated today, maybe, but that is probably all. Bring him along and we'll listen to his heart to make sure there are no arrhythmias or irregularities, but he should be fine.'

Mrs Bright was very relieved and promised to make sure it didn't happen again.

Mixing up medications is surprisingly common and invariably the owners are in a panic. Fortunately, it normally works out OK, but it needs an urgent vet call to double-check.

A more common problem with potentially very serious complications is when pets appear ill and are inappropriately given human medications by a member of the family in an attempt to help them. This is not recommended at all because many human medications are unsuitable for animals and can have serious, if not fatal, consequences. Paracetamol is a common example and must never ever be given to cats especially; the results are likely to be fatal.

Fortunately, the tablets involved in this case were relatively harmless for both Gyp and Mrs Bright. Phew!

Fair game

Brody was a five-year-old male beagle dog with a long history of visits to the veterinary clinic. Even as a pup his gastrointestinal system was challenged, and we had seen him multiple times for vomiting and diarrhoea.

He had always been a handful, and even at puppy school classes he pushed the boundaries. It was difficult for his owners, Kim and Neville, to control him, and he received more attention as a result and more training sessions. He responded, but then slipped back again as other priorities in life took over and training hours were reduced. On the other hand, he was a fun dog to have around and enjoyed the children's company, spending hours playing with them. The family loved him to bits, and they could dress him up or play tug of war with him.

As is often the case with these patients, multiple treatments had been tried. Some of them worked for a while, or were partially effective, only for Brodie to regress again after a period of treatment. Laboratory tests never really showed anything either. A low-fat and low-allergen diet seemed to help, but success never lasted.

Brody, like many of our patients, became more and more

anxious with repeat visits to the veterinary clinic. He was long-suffering, but moderately resistant to repeated and ongoing examinations. Each time he came in, he became more and more wound up. This would show as agitation, constant fretting and movement when I tried to examine him. It was all that Kim could do to hold him for an examination.

Quite often, he needed admission for the day to carry out laboratory tests, administer treatment and monitor his improvement or progress. At first, he was moderately OK when left at the clinic, with some initial, then intermittent periods of fretting. This generally involved pulling on the lead, jumping up or moving a lot when we tried to examine him or collect blood samples. It took several nurses to hold him or settle him. In his cage at the clinic he was not much better, pacing, ripping up his bedding and barking. As time went by, he got worse. Everything in his cage was shredded by teeth or paws. Sedation helped a little, but as he was often unwell, we did not want to overdo this. In the end, he had a big sign on his cage which read: 'ABSOLUTELY NOTHING IN CAGE – DESTROYS!'

The clinic had an array of cage warning signs or labels, some of which read: 'Owner only to remove from cage' (animal was aggressive), 'Care' (Bites), 'Extra Care' (Bites hard!), 'Vet ONLY to remove' (Bites really hard!), 'Escape Artist' (Escapes from cage if given a millimetre to wriggle through – believe me they are quick), 'Face Rubs' (Rubs face on the bars of the cage, removing the fur around their eyes and head!) With the face rubbers it is embarrassing to send cats home bald and owners are not happy, understandably. There was also an array of medical labels such as 'Nil By Mouth', 'Soft Food Only', 'Painful Injury', etc. We always administered sedation, if necessary, for anxiety or aggressiveness, and pain relief if and when needed. There were always new labels that needed to be created, as other needs arose.

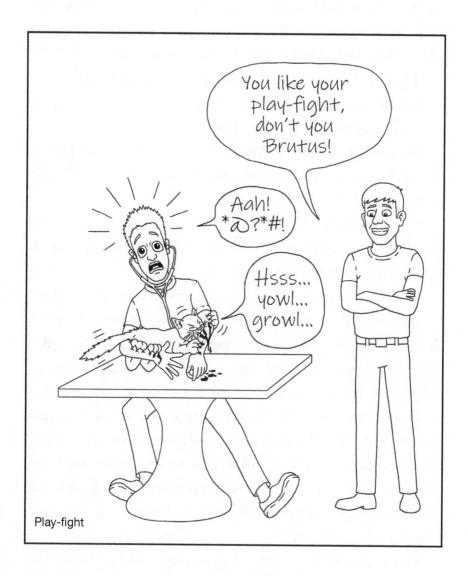
Play-fight

In Brody's case, it seemed that it took a huge dose of sedatives to settle him, so we tried to give priority to him, treat him early and send him home as soon as possible.

Kim had Brody booked in to see me again.

'Hello Kim, how are things going with Brody?' I asked.

'Well, Mike, not too good. Brody has lost one and a half kilograms of weight and his bowel is constantly upset now. It's quite a while since he has been normal. What are we going to do?'

'That's a shame, Kim. I think it's time to admit him and take some bowel samples and send them to the laboratory to help us get a firm diagnosis to help him here.'

'We have cost concerns, Mike; we only want to do that if it is absolutely necessary, as we can't afford it. Can you admit him, do some tests and then give me a call?'

'OK Kim, we'll admit him, run blood tests and take it from there,' I said, knowing that what he really needed was surgical biopsies, which they could not afford.

As time went by Brody was having more and more problems with his gut and now he was losing weight, so we didn't have any choice but to admit him and investigate further. We really needed to give him an anaesthetic and operate to collect biopsies, or samples of his gut, and send them for laboratory analysis. Tissue samples were often necessary to diagnose many disease conditions. Frequently, this was the only way to get an accurate diagnosis that would then allow you to administer the right treatment. Everyone is always very relieved and happy to know what the actual diagnosis is, because it allows us to target the most appropriate therapy.

Kim and Neville wanted a definite diagnosis for Brody. The time never seemed quite right financially, but would it ever be? We admitted Brody for blood tests and symptomatic treatment first to see how his blood protein levels and organ function were and if he improved with therapy for the day. On admission, he was blood tested and given medication after the usual battle. He was placed in a cage with absolutely nothing in it. Even metal water bowls were gnawed on repeatedly until they had dents in them or were otherwise demolished. His lead was hung on the outside of his cage door.

The blood results came through and they were normal. 'Well, that's great,' I said, and we decided on some appropriate symptomatic medication. I drew up the injections and we headed down to the dog kennels (Brody was kennelled as far away from earshot as possible to allow us some peace).

When we arrived, there was Brody in his cage with his stainless-steel chain-link lead now in the cage with him. He had pulled it in! But there was one problem. His chain-link lead had a looped leather handle that formed approximately half of the lead – or it did have. This was now nowhere to be seen. Lying on the floor of the cage was the length of chain-link with the dog clip on the end, but definitely no leather handle. A frantic search behind him and around the front of the cage produced nothing. Brody was not telling us where it was, but he was looking mighty pleased with himself. I turned to the nurse, Emma.

'Did that lead have a leather handle on it, or not?'

'Yep,' she said. There was no need for any further words.

'I didn't think I was going stupid,' I said.

There was only one explanation: Brody had eaten it.

The handle was wide and made of old, hard leather. Quite often when a dog eats something inappropriate (and this is common, as you might imagine) we give them a drug that makes them vomit, and up it comes a few minutes later. But this can only be done if what they have swallowed can be vomited without danger. That is, if it is sharp, hard, large, caustic, etc., then to make them vomit would potentially do more harm than good as it may well damage tissues on the way back up or worse, get stuck. The leather handle fitted that description, so it would have to be removed surgically.

I rang Kim and Neville.

'Hello Kim, it's Mike here. Brody is fine. There are two lots of news to report to you [in other words, there is good and bad news]. The blood tests were normal, and I have administered some medication. The other news is that he has chewed up and swallowed the leather handle of his lead and he needs surgery to remove it! But Kim, in a way this is good news because while we're in there to remove the leather handle from his stomach we can take several biopsies from different areas of his gut to get a definitive diagnosis. This is what he needs.'

Kim was very happy to have biopsies taken as part of the unexpected surgery that needed doing at the same time.

Fortunately, the surgery went well, and the biopsies told us that Brody had an immune mediated bowel condition. This meant that when Brody had recovered from the surgery, we were able to start appropriate and targeted treatment, to which we got a reasonably good response.

From then on, if Brody had to stay at the clinic in a cage, his sign read:

'ABSOLUTELY NOTHING IN OR HANGING ON CAGE.'

Needle in a haystack

German shepherd dogs have consistently been a popular dog through the years that I have been a practising veterinarian. Like all large-breed dogs, they have their share of health problems. Hip and elbow dysplasia are much more common in large-breed dogs, but breeders can reduce the incidence of this by scoring their breeding dogs and selecting dogs with lower scores to breed from. Specific breed-related health conditions also occur in the German shepherd and many can be well managed, in general, with the advanced drugs that are available nowadays. There is still a lot to learn, though, and research is ongoing.

The phone rang. 'Hello, it's Robyn, Jodi's mum here. He's just swallowed a needle; I'm rushing him down.'

And with that the phone line went dead and Jodi's panicked mum was making a beeline for the clinic! We all knew who Jodi and Robyn were, so there was no need for surnames or further details

Jodi had a bad start to life and had lost one of his eyes as the result of an unfortunate incident. He had been 'rescued' and, with lots of TLC in his new home, had grown into a fine dog. The name Jodi is very sentimental: 'Jo' comes from one of the rescue agency's dedicated foster mums, who had sadly passed away at a relatively young age, and 'di' is part of his new mum's name. He certainly was spirited and full of life, a very fitting tribute to his namesakes.

Jodi had a pretty good life though. Robyn, his mum, was a dedicated German shepherd owner of many years so understood the breed well and the specific breed-related health issues they can suffer from. In saying that, Jodi was a healthy dog and was not afflicted with any of these health concerns, yet!

Unusually, Jodi had decided to grab a needle with thread attached and swallow it! Robyn had seen him take it into his mouth and had rushed over only to see him swallow it! This is often the case when the canine culprit tries to get whatever they have grabbed down into their stomach without delay. As dog owners, many of us have seen this on numerous occasions while walking our own dogs when they grab discarded delicacies like chicken bones or bread. When Robyn opened Jodi's mouth to see if she could retrieve the needle and thread all she could see was the end of the pink thread. The attached needle was presumably further down the oesophagus making its way to the stomach.

They soon arrived and there was no sign of the needle or thread now. Presumably, they had moved further down into Jodi's stomach. Robyn was adamant they had not come out of Jodi's mouth as she had been with him the whole time.

'Well, Robyn, we had better take an X-ray and see if the needle is visible.'

Although a needle is thin, it is stainless steel and therefore radio-dense, which means it will show up as a reasonably strong white colour on our radiographs, or X-rays. This is useful if you are looking for a foreign body, as in this case, or monitoring healing after implanting stainless-steel or titanium bone implants.

As Jodi was nearly fifty kilograms, he needed some chemical restraint to allow us to X-ray him, so we administered a sedative. Once the sedative had taken effect, we opened his mouth and, no, there was no sign of the needle or thread. We aligned the X-ray cone and stepped back with our lead aprons, gloves, and neck protectors on to shield us from the scattered X-ray beams and took the X-ray. Digital X-ray processors nowadays make life a lot simpler and a minute or so after inserting the X-ray cassette into the processor – there it was on the screen – a long thin needle in the stomach. There was no doubting it and Jodi's owner Robyn was not surprised.

'Well, where else is it going to be?' she proclaimed. 'I saw him swallow it.'

She was right and thank goodness it was in the stomach and not stuck in the oesophagus, which runs through the chest cavity. That would have been another story.

'Yes, you're right, Robyn, where else is it going to be? Well, we are going to have to do some surgery – a laparotomy to be precise, which involves opening the abdominal cavity. Then we will need to do a gastrostomy, or opening of the stomach, to locate the needle, remove it and suture everything closed.'

'You'd better get on with it then, hadn't you,' were her pragmatic words. Robyn knew the drill.

So, we put Jodi back in his cage and set up for the surgical procedure. We then took him out to the toilet before inserting an intravenous catheter and starting him on intravenous fluids. He was a big dog and only just fitted in our surgery cages. He was still feeling a bit groggy from our sedation which premedicated him well for the surgery. After a while we gave him the full general anaesthetic and prepared him for surgery.

After lifting him through into the sterile theatre room and disinfecting his clipped skin, we draped his abdomen and performed the celiotomy (an incision in the abdomen). We opened his stomach and started to explore for the needle. A pair of long thin sterile forceps inserted into the stomach should have been able to grab the offending needle as it is metal and hard, quite different to the soft movable stomach wall. The stomach appeared empty and we still could not find any needle. This was unusual. We had a discussion and thought it a good idea to extend the length of the incision in the stomach wall so we could explore better and shine a surgical light inside. I even placed my sterile gloved hand into the stomach to have a gentle feel around. To my surprise and horror there appeared to be no needle! This was most odd. Maybe it had already moved into the small intestine?

With this in mind we sutured the stomach closed and flushed the area with sterile warm saline and set about inspecting the small bowel. Initially, we looked at the proximal or first part, with no luck. We should have been able to feel a hard straight needle through the intestinal wall, but no, there was no needle to feel. As we progressed along the entire length of the small bowel there was still no sign of the needle. How could this be? After all, we had seen it clearly on the X-ray maybe an hour or two earlier.

Now, the small bowel runs into the large bowel via a junction where the remnants of the caecum, or appendix, is. There was no sign here either and we had a feel as far as we could through the large bowel – still no needle. How could a sharp thin needle that was at risk of perforating the bowel travel this far anyway, and in only a couple of hours. Not possible, I thought.

We had another look through the bowel and again found nothing.

It would have been handy to have had fluoroscopy. This is a medical imaging machine that shows an X-ray on a monitor in real-time so you can use it during surgery. It is very expensive and mainly used in human hospitals and by specialists, so alas, we did not have it.

Where could the needle have gone? We knew it had made it to the stomach. But if it were not there, what else could we do? So, we sutured Jodi closed, then carried him through and took another X-ray. There it was, but now it appeared as though it might be in the large bowel or colon! How the heck did it get there so quickly?

We woke Jodi up and had a discussion with Robyn. We advised Robyn that he may pass the needle, as it was now in his colon, which is much wider and full of semisolid content. Foreign bodies, if they make it to the large bowel or colon, are often passed from the body with no problem. If they are in the small bowel or intestine, they are much more likely to cause an obstruction or perforate the bowel.

No one could explain its location. But there it was on the X-ray after the surgery for all to see.

It was not long after Jodi had arrived home that he had several good bowel movements and Robyn discovered the needle in one of them. She was overjoyed when she rang with the good news, and so were we, but we are still scratching our heads over this one.

Interestingly, on numerous occasions over the years I have seen cases where animals have swallowed pieces of jewellery, including wedding rings. The normal procedure if the dog is a medium to large breed, is to wait. All things will pass! Normally within twenty-four hours, not two hours, the item is passed, everyone is happy, and the valuable or sentimental item is carefully washed and returned to the rightful owner.

How long?

Animals, being mammals, have a body system that functions in a very similar way to humans'. There are some notable anatomical or structural differences, and this is fascinating to study as a veterinary student, although there is plenty to remember.

Sheep, cows, goats, and deer are foregut fermenters and have four chambers to their stomachs, the first two are fermenting vats that break down the cellulose in grass so it can be processed and absorbed further on. Horses, rabbits, rats, koalas and rhinoceros are hindgut fermenters, which means the fermenting vat is at the end of the small intestine, not the beginning. Humans have just the one stomach and cannot digest the cellulose in grass. There are numerous other structural differences, especially in large animals. Examples include that the horse at birth has one toe – the hoof – and the horse and other large animals have a 'stay apparatus' or an accumulation of muscles, ligaments and tendons that effectively locks legs allowing them to enter a light sleep while standing, and not fall over! Interestingly, I talked earlier about the bone in the dog's penis, the os penis, and the glans penis, which can result in tying while mating.

Although many mammals have anal glands, those of cats and dogs seem to be more developed. They are located at four and eight o'clock just inside the anus in these species and function as scent-marking glands. Most pet owners are aware of these structures, especially as they can cause problems that often result in a visit to the vet.

As an animal ages these glands can occasionally become cancerous; again, this is more frequently seen in dogs.

Jed was an eleven-year-old desexed male golden retriever dog. He belonged to an elderly gentleman, Mr Bristol. Like most golden retrievers, Jed was a very happy-go-lucky dog that was everyone's friend, as evidenced by his constantly wagging tail. He loved visits to the vet clinic and especially the treats that the nurses had for him! His owner, Mr Bristol, was a character. His manner was brusque and to the point, he did not pull any punches, so to speak, and at times this came across as bordering on rude. However, Mr Bristol was always grateful and thankful for good service when he got it and was a loyal, faithful client. Once you got to know him, he was a very affable character, but certainly not one to take lightly. His communication style was a series of short sharp military-style probing questions and once he was satisfied with the response you knew you had won him over and you could relax, a little.

We had not seen Jed for a while, but he still made a beeline for the counter as usual and the treats, as soon as he entered the door. He was not disappointed, but there was always room for more.

'Hello, Mr Bristol, how are you today?'

'It's my dog I've come about. I will let you know when you've told me what the problem is,' he replied.

'OK, well let's go through and examine him.'

Jed headed for the consulting room looking for more treats, so we didn't disappoint him. Once in there, Mr Bristol did not waste time before explaining. 'It's his rear end I want you to look at today. Looks like there's a swelling there and he's straining to defecate a bit too,' he said.

Not wanting to waste time, I proceeded to examine the affected area straight away.

'Yes, I can feel a lump on the right side of his anus, Mr Bristol. I'll just put a glove on and examine it further.'

'Well, what's the story then?'

There was a sense of urgency now as I had confirmed his suspicions, and he needed to know.

'It is quite hard so it could be a tumour.'

'What, cancer? Is that what you mean?'

'It could be, yes. I'll just examine the area further.'

I wanted to make sure that it was not an abscess or some other form of cellulitis, but it did feel ominous.

I put a rectal glove on with some lubricant and had a gentle feel inside the anus along the rectal canal. I could feel that the lump was very hard and about three to four centimetres long by one and a half centimetres wide. The gland on the other side though, was normal. Better not to delay the discussion any further.

'Mr Bristol, it is probably a cancerous growth, yes, and most likely an anal gland adenocarcinoma, or tumour of the right anal gland.'

'Hmph, well what are you going to do about it? Cut it out I suppose.'

'Yes, that's the best plan. But we'll need to do some blood

tests first to check organ function and blood calcium level amongst other things.'

'Well, when can you do it? Can you do it now?'

'We'll take some bloods now and provisionally book Jed in for surgery tomorrow, Mr Bristol.'

It was best to attend to Jed straight away, and luckily, we had time tomorrow. Mr Bristol was not happy to wait once a problem was identified.

So off he went with Jed, to return tomorrow.

Anal gland adenocarcinoma, once found, needs to be surgically removed if possible. There are certain characteristics that determine the prognosis. If the animal is well, blood calcium level normal, and the tumour small, with no signs of spread, it is better. Luckily for Jed, the calcium was normal, he seemed well, but the tumour was of moderate size. The larger it is the more likely it has spread to the local lymph glands and beyond. Also, a large growth is more difficult to remove with clean margins, that is, enough surrounding normal tissue. The bigger the clean margin, the less likely it is to grow back.

The next day the surgery went well for Jed, but the lump was a reasonable size and I was worried about it returning in the future. As there are some essential structures in that area, such as the anal sphincter and the rectum, these must be carefully identified and preserved. Therefore, you cannot remove much surrounding normal-looking tissue.

We sent the growth off to the diagnostic laboratory and waited for the result.

When it came back, unfortunately it confirmed our suspicions.

Mr Bristol did not want any follow up chemotherapy or specialist treatment, so we used some anti-inflammatory medication which might help prevent the regrowth and keep Jed comfortable, for now. Mr Bristol wanted to know how long Jed had. I gave him a range of survival times according to the published data but let him know it was difficult to predict.

We scheduled check-ups to assess for any regrowth.

It was about eight to ten months later when Mr Bristol finally came back for a check-up for Jed. The tumour was re-growing, and it was quite big already and would be impossible to remove successfully. Second surgeries were often difficult, and generally did not achieve as much, apart from temporarily debulking or reducing the size of the tumour.

'How long's he got?' was one of the first questions Mr Bristol asked at the revisit.

This was understandable, but it is difficult to say because it depended on a lot of factors and varied between patients.

'It can vary, Mr Bristol; it could be months or longer.'

'Yes, but how long has he got? One month, three months, how long?'

Mr Bristol was quite determined to get an estimate out of me.

'I can't be sure now, Mr Bristol, but it will probably be several months.'

'Hmph, not long then,' he exclaimed.

'It is difficult to say; it's just an estimate.'

Off he went with further check-ups scheduled and a discussion about what to look out for if there were going to be any problems. We kept Jed on anti-inflammatory medication to possibly help slow the regrowth and keep him comfortable. More pain relief and symptomatic treatment could be added in, as needed.

After several months it appeared that Jed's regrowth rate was slow, and he was doing well.

About four months after I had discovered the regrowth, Mr Bristol was sitting in the waiting room chatting with several other clients when I overheard him announcing to the assembled gathering: 'This is the dog that Mr Small said would only live a couple of months!'

My ears pricked up a bit. It was only four months and I had been very careful to say it was very hard to predict survival rates!

'Come on in, Mr Bristol, thanks.'

In bounced Jed with Mr Bristol in tow and he was looking good. The tumour was re-growing slowly but steadily but otherwise he seemed in good health. We took a blood sample to check organ function and his blood count, dispensing some more anti-inflammatory pain-relief medication.

'Jed's doing well, that's a good sign. That's very pleasing.'

'Hmph, yeah, and you said he would only live a couple of months.'

'Well the longer the better, Mr Bristol. This is pleasing. Remember it is difficult to predict, as I said, and it varies between patients from a few months to more. We just don't know. As long as he's comfortable and happy that's the main thing.'

'When will I see you again?' he asked.

'Maybe every one to two months for a check-up and more medication.'

'That often?'

'It would be a good idea so I can adjust any medication and keep an eye on his organ function and calcium levels and any obstruction developing in his anal area.'

With that Mr Bristol departed.

Every time Mr Bristol came in, the same announcement was made to the assembled and receptive audience in the waiting room. 'This is the dog that Mr Small said would only live a couple of months!' As time went on, it became more elaborate and convincing and the audience more enraptured.

I made a mental note to be very careful in the future about being pushed for such predictions. Selective memory is a convenient thing!

Jed lived for about a year before, sadly, we had to make the decision to euthanise him.

Double bolt

My first ten years in veterinary practice were split between farm calls and small-animal practice. This made for a varied working life in two quite different worlds, the clinic, and then the very scenic drives out to farms, with some trepidation if the weather was bad and I had an outdoor job to do, or it involved unpredictable animals such as large stags. These powerful animals could be very unfriendly, but normally I could sedate them quickly before they lashed out . . . but not always! You certainly stayed away from any that had hard antler on them during the mating season, a time when they were particularly unfriendly. In fact, the hinds (female deer) often lashed out more. Once, when a hind reared up and raked my hand, inflicting a nasty gash, I needed a row of sutures afterwards. I have had to retreat over the fence on several occasions when chased out of a paddock. If there is any doubt, it is best to hug the fence line, or not go in in the first place!

One of the common large-animal surgical procedures I performed, although sporadically, was gelding a male horse. This is necessary to make them easier to handle and reduce their sex drive. Generally, only valuable stud stallions are left entire for breeding purposes. Gelding is undertaken in a pen, a yard or a paddock. It is preferable to have a soft clean area of grass as it is often performed under a general anaesthetic. In a general mixed practice like we had, gelding was not a big part of the practice, unlike in some large horse-only practices where it is a more common procedure. In these practices I have seen it done while the horse is standing with sedation, pain relief and local anaesthesia, but you need good facilities and experience. Sometimes there is no suitable yard, so if the horse is amenable, the procedure can be undertaken in a paddock. Most farmers and experienced horse owners are good at handling and restraining their animals for the veterinarian.

It is well known in veterinary circles that while some lifestyle or hobby farms have good facilities or yards – indeed some of them can resemble Fort Knox – many more do not have good yards. Often, if they exist at all, they are a ramshackle Heath-Robinson affair, only high enough for sheep and not cattle or horses. Or worse still, the yards are dilapidated! I have seen all sorts of arrangements and have spent many hours trying to get an animal, or animals, into the yards, and then trying to examine and treat patients in ramshackle yards. Sometimes, you just give up and go to plan B another day. It can appear very funny to bystanders, watching a circus act taking place before their eyes, but it's not always so much fun for those involved!

On this day, though, we were out in the country air, in a paddock.

Rick Hughes had rung up the week before and booked his stallion, Heck, in for gelding on the Wednesday. He had been doing some training with him, but he was becoming increasingly difficult to handle, and it was time for the chop.

You need a fine day for this procedure, and favourable weather. Wednesday morning had dawned a bit stormy, so, I rang Rick.

'Hello Rick, Mike Small here, how are you?'

'All good, Doc, thanks. You still coming up?'

'Yes, provided the weather's going to be OK.'

'Should be all right. It's supposed to cut up later, but the job will be over by then.'

He also had a horse cover he would place on Heck after we gelded him.

'OK, Rick, I'll be up shortly.'

With that, I loaded up the car and headed out to Rick's farm.

When I arrived, the skies were looking a bit grey and ominous, but there was no rain, so we had a window in which to geld Heck and allow him to recover before the weather turned.

Once you have made an appointment, put the time aside, assembled your equipment and sterilised it, driven the distance to the farm – often quite a distance! – there is a lot more pressure to see the job through. Not at all costs, though, but often you will push things a little. This might be the case today, I thought.

'OK, Rick, let's get to it,' I said.

Heck was a little jumpy, but Rick was a good horse handler.

I sedated Heck and we waited a few minutes for that to take effect. Meanwhile, I laid out the surgical kit and got the intravenous anaesthetic ready.

If I was to do a more involved procedure like a longer stitch-up – for example, when horses got caught in barbed-wire fences and injured themselves and needed multiple sutures – then I would put an intravenous catheter in the jugular vein in the neck and infuse a muscle relaxant and anaesthetic combination and the horse would gradually become anaesthetised. You can then give top-up doses through the indwelling catheter you have in the neck to keep them anaesthetised.

At that time, when I gave the anaesthetic to castrate a horse, it was delivered as a concentrated solution of short-acting anaesthetic into the jugular vein in the neck. The knock-down dose was administered quickly before the needle was withdrawn and we steadied the horse as it keeled over a few seconds later. You had to be quick otherwise you might not get the full dose in before he started to go down. If you did not get the full dose in quickly, they might not get enough and you had to try to get the vein once they relaxed and get more anaesthetic in; not an ideal situation. Worse still was when you only got a little in and they went into the excitement phase of anaesthesia! You normally avoid this by giving a reasonable dose quickly into the vein and they pass through this phase undetected on the way to full anaesthetic relaxation.

Heck appeared reasonably sedated, which was good.

The weather was starting to close in as I inserted the needle into the neck, with Rick steadying Heck, and I thought I had better make it quick.

I then attached the syringe to the needle and drew back on the syringe to check I was still in the vein.

As I started to inject the anaesthetic there was a flash of lightning that shot across the sky. I continued to quickly inject the remaining anaesthetic as an almighty clap of thunder resounded through the air and a low rumble followed.

Heck reared up and shot across the paddock at full speed before eventually collapsing in a heap, anaesthetised!

I grabbed my sterile gear, which I had laid out neatly on the ground, and we sprinted across to Heck where he had collapsed. We hastily prepared him for the surgery and gelded him.

It was probably just as well we were in a paddock and fortunate we were standing some distance away from any fences, especially barbed-wire ones. To this day I can still see Heck belting off across the paddock.

His recovery was less eventful. It had been a close call, and I decided to geld any future patients only on fine days.

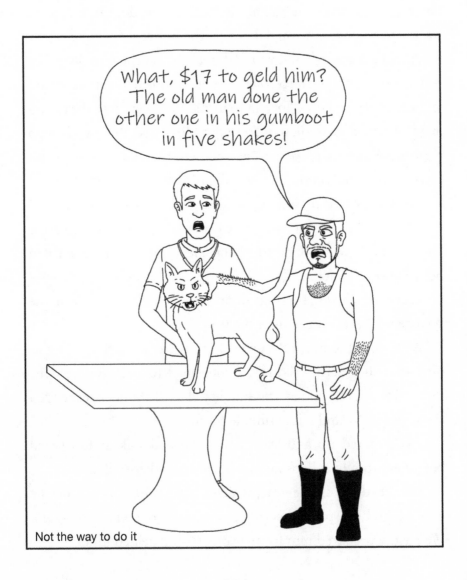

Not the way to do it

Watch that puppy

Poppy was a four-month-old shih-tzu-cross puppy who was normally very energetic, like most puppies. She was a real character and loved to play with her toys, and she already had a huge collection. She belonged to a young couple who doted on her, although we had not seen much of them lately and she was overdue for her second puppy vaccination.

My nurse Debbie came out to the surgery and informed me that Mic and Sarah had been on the phone concerned about their pup. She seemed quite lethargic this morning. They had had a party the night before and were worried she had grabbed something she shouldn't have, or she had been fed something that had upset her.

'Debbie, tell them to come on down. That doesn't sound right. Poppy will need a check-up,' I said.

Debbie organised an appointment in half an hour's time. I finished my surgery and made my way to the waiting room. Just as I entered it, Mic and Sarah arrived. They looked a bit dishevelled and I decided it must have been a good party the night before, and today would be a slow day for them.

'Come on through,' I said as I motioned them into the consulting room.

Poppy was in a blanket and was certainly looking out of sorts.

'Poppy certainly doesn't look her normal self today. What's the story?'

They waited for each other to speak and eventually Mic spoke.

'We're not sure, but we had a few friends around last night for some drinks and food. She was all right then, but maybe she grabbed something, and she's got food poisoning or something.'

'Have there been any other symptoms apart from this lethargy?' I asked.

Poppy was just lying there on her blanket semi-conscious and her pupils looked a bit dilated. The blanket she was lying on was wet under her mouth so it appeared she might be drooling saliva.

'No,' was the reply. There was not any other information forthcoming, so I thought I had better examine her and see what I could find. Maybe they were a bit hungover or tired themselves; they certainly looked it.

I examined her all over. I could see her pupils were moderately dilated, she was quite limp and non-responsive and if you lifted her up, she flopped down again and could hardly stand. I listened to her chest. Her heart and respiratory rate seemed a bit low. I could not find anything of note in her abdomen on palpation. Her temperature was not elevated and, if anything, it was a little low, which would fit with her level of consciousness.

'Has there been any vomiting or diarrhoea?' I asked.

'No.'

'Any falls? Did someone drop her?'

'No.'

Mmm, all a bit unusual. Obviously, I had not found too much

apart from a sleepy, depressed pup, but there were concerning slight decreases in her vital signs and her nervous system seemed a bit depressed.

'We need to keep Poppy in the hospital and run blood tests to check her organ function, blood-glucose level and blood count. It would be a good idea to put her on intravenous fluids, give her some glucose and try to warm her. We will need to closely monitor her vital signs every hour or so to make sure they do not worsen. Hopefully, they will improve with the supportive treatment. We do not have a lot more to go on at this point. Maybe ask around your friends who were there last night to see if they noticed anything unusual and give us a call if you think of anything else please.'

I was scratching my head a bit but maybe the blood test would show something. If it did not, it was a matter of wait and see and monitor.

With that, Mic and Sarah left. Maybe they would come up with more information, I thought.

We gave Poppy fluids and warmed her. She still seemed sleepy but her vital signs did not deteriorate, so it was just a waiting game.

The blood test results were unremarkable for a young pup. We took a screening X-ray in case there was anything else of note in her chest or abdominal cavity. But we could see nothing there either.

We were standing looking at Poppy when a thought occurred to us.

What sort of party was it? Who was there, and what were they doing?

I thought I had better ring Mic and Sarah and ask further questions.

'Hi Mic, it's Mike here, the vet. Poppy is doing OK, a little bit better, her temperature has come up a little and her blood test and X-ray did not show anything of concern. But I have to ask a couple of questions and, if you don't mind, I'd appreciate a straight answer please. Don't be offended but I have to ask this in Poppy's interest. Is there any chance Poppy could have eaten a weed brownie, or marijuana cookie, or something like that?'

There was a long silence on the end of the phone.

'Hello, Mic, are you there?'

'Yep, I'm here.'

'I think that is what Poppy is suffering from. It just fits. If someone had some weed or similar and she grabbed it – it could explain what happened to her. Is that correct?'

After another pause there was a brief response. 'Well I suppose it's possible.'

'OK, that's good to know, so someone had some, eh, and maybe she grabbed some and ate it. I reckon that's it . . . Do you agree?'

'Yeah probably.'

That was all I needed to know. Sometimes these things are better winkled out of an owner over the phone. They are not face to face with you and all they need to do is say nothing, agree or disagree. Generally, saying nothing or agreeing is a positive. It is less likely there will be a firm denial if it's put to them that way and they know it's likely.

We gave Poppy charcoal to help limit any further absorption of the weed, although it was probably a bit late by now. She would just have to sleep it off.

Animals are quite sensitive to the effects of marijuana, more so than humans, and especially a young small-breed puppy.

Firstly, their weight is lower so not much drug is needed to have an effect, and secondly, young animals are more sensitive to drugs as their metabolising pathways in the liver are not as well developed. Also, for Poppy, she was very energetic, so she was quite lean which made her more sensitive, too. It was lucky she did not eat more than she did because the effects can be life-threatening.

Later that day Poppy was starting to lift her head and she showed some interest in food and soon ate a lot. By the next day she was more like the old Poppy, and certainly she was ready to go home later that day.

Next time they had a party they would make sure Poppy was watched and had been well fed beforehand.

Sleeping dogs don't tell

Some people are cat people, others prefer dogs, however a lot of clients have both cats and dogs. But it can be double trouble! It is amazing how often cats just turn up on doorsteps and that's it, they have a home for life. Sometimes, it seemed about twenty to thirty per cent of our clients acquired their felines this way. Whether it is a neighbour's cat that prefers life on the other side of the fence, or a dumped kitten – which, unfortunately, happens too often – they know when they've found a loving home and you've got a new family member for life. Cats are usually independent characters and can be left to their own devices. They eat and entertain themselves periodically and sleep the rest of the day. This suits many people's lifestyles . . . they don't have to be home all day.

Dogs, on the other hand, require constant company and prefer someone home all day, such as a family or retired couple, or someone who works from home. Most of the behavioural problems we see can either be traced to poor upbringing or training, or separation anxiety problems. There are many reasons why you cannot leave a dog at home all day, not least is the need for constant company and someone to take them out for exercise. Walks once or twice daily keep everyone fit.

The Watsons were longstanding clients who came in periodically with their family pets. There had been a succession of both cats and dogs over the years. Like any large family, there was a lot of activity and the inevitable incidents and accidents from time to time.

They had unfortunately very recently lost both their cat and dog due to age-related health problems. This is not an uncommon situation when pets are acquired at a similar time and age together. Of course, many cats outlive dogs, as normally cats live for longer.

Recently the Watsons had acquired a four-month-old labrador puppy and named him Basil. I am not sure if it was after Basil Brush, but maybe not, because Basil was a fox! The family was very happy with Basil and loved him to bits. He was like all puppies, though, and especially labrador puppies – very mischievous and keen to chew on everything in sight.

The Watsons were not very happy this morning. They had rung up very upset a short time earlier and were on their way down to the clinic, with Basil. They had woken in the morning to find Basil lying on the floor beside his basket unresponsive. He was still breathing, but he appeared unconscious, or asleep. They could not rouse him, which, for a normally exuberant puppy, was most unusual and very concerning.

They soon arrived and the family rushed in with Basil in a basket. We hurried them into the examination room, and they congregated around the table looking expectantly at me for answers.

'Hello everyone, any idea what happened to Basil?'

'No, no, none at all. We woke this morning and there he was

lying next to his basket just as you see him now. He seemed OK last night.'

'Did he eat his normal dinner last night?' I asked.

'Yes, yes he did.'

'Anything else happen?'

'No.'

I thought I had better get straight to work examining Basil without asking any more questions as there was a sense of great urgency here, and rightly so.

I lifted his head gently and there were no reflexes present, and no jaw tone. In other words, there was no eye-blink reflex and I could open his mouth and he would not bite down at all. I gently placed his head back on the blanket. His limbs were flaccid, and there was no withdrawal of his limbs to pinch pressure on his toes. His breathing was slow and regular. His heart rate and body temperature were lower than normal, and he was unconscious. At least he didn't have a rapid, pounding heart or laboured breathing, which could indicate a more serious problem. But he was depressed for sure, and asleep.

Now this reminded me ominously of the case of Poppy and the marijuana, but the Watsons? This family certainly did not look like they would have drugs in the house, but you can never assume anything.

I had to broach the subject but, with the whole family present, I had to be careful.

'Are there any prescription medicines or other drugs in the house, on the bedside cabinet or in the bathroom cabinet that Basil could get into and swallow that would send him off to sleep like this?' I asked. That, I thought, was a better way to phrase the question to a family.

A thoughtful look came over the face of Brian, the dad. But it was not long before he said, 'No, not at all, nothing left out, and nothing like that in our house anyway.'

'He hasn't had any falls or accidents, or run onto the road?' I knew this was a long shot because Basil did not appear to have any injuries or signs of trauma.

'No, not at all, our section is fenced. Kids, do you know of anything? Did anyone drop him or step on him? He didn't fall off the deck or anything?'

They all shook their heads. Nobody had anything to report.

I had a look at him again. He was a little dirty and muddy, but it was winter, and he had probably been out in the backyard.

'Look, everyone, we'll admit Basil and run blood tests and take an X-ray to see what we can find. We'll put him on intravenous fluids and warm him up to increase his body temperature. It's a bit low. I'll let you know what we find. There's not much more we can do at the moment, but he seems stable enough at this point,' I said.

He was breathing slowly but rhythmically, and his mucous membrane colour was a nice healthy pink.

With that, they left a little reluctantly, still searching my face for answers which I could not give at this point. I was scratching my head as much as they were and could only think there were some similarities to Poppy's case earlier in the week, but this family was different. The Watsons had not held a party, nor baked hash cookies, well, not as far as we knew anyway, but it was very unlikely! Normally I'd expect to see some other symptoms if the puppy had eaten something toxic and there were no obvious ones. We would just have to wait, treat any symptoms and see if our tests showed anything helpful.

So, we connected the intravenous drip and pump to Basil, took blood and put him on a heat pad and wrapped him up. We waited for the blood results, which did not take long to process. When they came through, there was nothing to note apart from a mild electrolyte imbalance. Mmm, more head-scratching.

We had better take an X-ray, I thought. It probably would not show us anything, but you never knew.

We took a screening X-ray and apart from evidence of a bony meal having been eaten recently we could not see anything. Maybe they were feeding a raw bony diet.

I rang the Watsons to report.

'Hello Brian. Basil is stable on the drip and is warming up a bit with the heat pad and blankets and warm intravenous fluids. His breathing is OK. His blood test came back fairly normal. The X-ray ... there is nothing much to see. What do you feed Basil?'

'He gets puppy biscuits and canned food.'

'OK. That sounds good. Do you feed him bones as well?' I wasn't that keen on owners feeding a young dog like this bones but now wasn't the time to drill them on it!

'No, no, not at all. One of my previous dogs had a problem with bones and constipation, so I won't feed them.'

'That's a bit odd, Brian. There are some bones in his stomach. Has any of the family fed him bones? Any of the kids, or your wife?'

'Not that I know of, but I'll check.'

Brian went off and asked the family and it was not long before he was back on the phone.

'No, nobody has fed him any bones.'

'Does he wander off your section, Brian?'

'No, he can't, it's fenced.'

'Look, hang on Brian, I'll have another look at the X-ray,' I said.

Was I seeing things? I had to double-check.

So, I went and had another look at the X-ray image on the screen.

Yes, there were definitely bones in there, and there were quite a few when I looked harder.

It was then that I saw it . . . Could it be? But why would it . . . ?

Then the penny dropped.

'Brian, can you put the phone down and go into your back yard and have a look please. Has Basil been digging there?'

'OK, will do.' Off he went to have a look.

It was not long before he was back.

He picked up the phone:

'Yes, there's a large hole there—'

I knew what the next words would be.

'He's gone and dug up poor old Sooty and . . . '

That was all I needed to hear.

Just two weeks ago we had euthanised the family cat of eighteen years, Sooty. Brian and Sandy had taken him home and buried him in the backyard. Unfortunately, Basil had been left alone for a period in the backyard and had dug him up and consumed not only Sooty, but a good dose of the pentobarbital, or barbiturate, used to euthanise him.

Fortunately, Basil made a good recovery. I am not so sure the family recovered as quickly, though. Since then, I always stress the need to bury family pets at home deeply.

It only happens to a vet

The following scenario has probably played out more often than we think over the years. Vets believe that it's never ever going to happen to them of course, because they always check and double-check. But the reality is, that some days are just so frantic that a comedy of errors can add up to a mistake. Fortunately, it can normally be corrected, and that is the important thing, never mind the embarrassment and need for profuse apologies.

The phone rang and it was Joanne Wilks.

'Hello, is that the vet clinic?'

'Yes, how can I help you today?'

'I'd like to book Thelma in for desexing.'

'No problem Joanne, how about this Thursday?'

Thelma, a six-month-old black and white female cat, was duly booked in to be spayed.

On Thursday there was a lot of surgery to get through and Thelma was admitted, checked over by the vet and a premedication, or sedation, given before the anaesthetic. Half an hour or so later Thelma was given a full anaesthetic and the nurse clipped her abdomen to prepare her for spaying. Thelma then had her

236

abdomen carefully disinfected before she was moved through to surgery where the vet, who had scrubbed up, put on sterile surgical gloves and a gown. A sterile drape was laid over Thelma, an incision made, and the abdomen explored in the quest for Thelma's uterine horns.

The problem was, the uterus could not be found, no matter how hard we tried.

The answer was that Thelma was in fact a male cat. Unfortunate Thelma then had 'her' abdomen sutured closed. Then, the scrotum at Thelma's back end under the tail below the anus was clipped and surgically prepared and the relatively simple procedure of castration completed. No abdomen needed to be opened for this procedure.

Profuse apologies followed, generally with no charge for the abdominal surgery, only a cat castration was charged for.

When I have seen this happen the client has always been very understanding. Fortunately. It only happens to a vet once! The moral of the story is: Always check the sex of an animal before you desex, no matter their name.

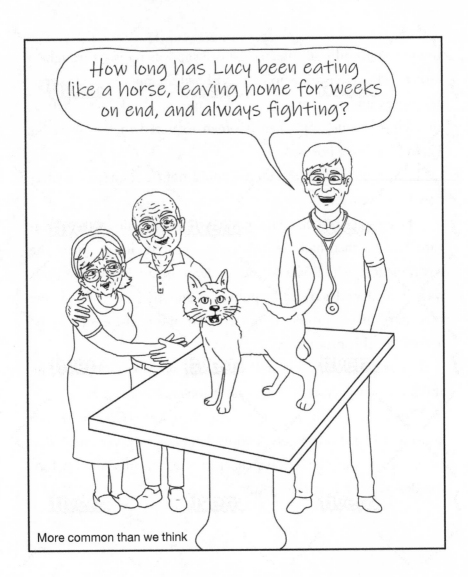

More common than we think

Spring gain

It was late spring when I saw Lulu, a young domestic short-hair tortoiseshell female cat with her very concerned owners, Wilma and Ed. The owner thought Lulu was about one year old but that was an estimate, as it often is. Lulu had turned up one day as a stray kitten, in very poor condition. It was likely she had been dumped by someone as she seemed friendly enough and had obviously had human contact, but her growth was stunted. She did have a big flea and worm burden, which was successfully treated. Not long after this she developed ringworm of her skin, which was also successfully treated. Poor Lulu. But she now had a loving home and had rapidly gained condition, making up for her poor start in life. We had not seen Lulu for many months, and she certainly had improved dramatically and responded to the tender loving care of Wilma and Ed Brunton. This type of story is much more common than you think and in fact a large number of our feline patients have had a bad beginning. Most of them quickly adapt to their new home and almost always flourish.

This was certainly the case with Lulu. She was the first cat that Wilma and Ed had owned so it was a learning curve for them.

'How are you, Wilma ... Ed?' I asked. 'We haven't seen you for a while.'

As they walked into the examination room Wilma looked very worried.

'I'm very concerned about Lulu, Mr Small. All of a sudden she has gained a lot of weight and she's eating so much. I'm worried she has a cancerous growth in her or some other disease. Maybe I'm just overfeeding her. It's not normal, and we should have brought her in to see you sooner but it's the finances you know, we're just pensioners. I feel so guilty, I hope she's OK.'

Wilma lifted the cat box and I could see her struggling to put it on the examination table so I helped, and yes, the weight inside the box was significant. Wilma lifted the lid and out hopped Lulu. I could see she had a very swollen abdomen.

'See what I mean, Mr Small? That's not normal is it? What could it be do you think?'

Now I had an idea, looking at her, but I thought it best to wait until I had some further information from my clinical examination. I gently palpated Lulu's abdomen, and this added weight to my suspicions. I had a look under Lulu's tummy and palpated gently. Lulu did not seem to mind any of this and was very smoochy and amorous.

'Well Wilma, you can relax, it's nothing serious. Lulu is pregnant. She's gaining weight because she has at least four kittens on board – she may have more – but I can feel four in her belly at least.'

'Really, Mr Small? I'm so relieved. I never would have imagined ... '

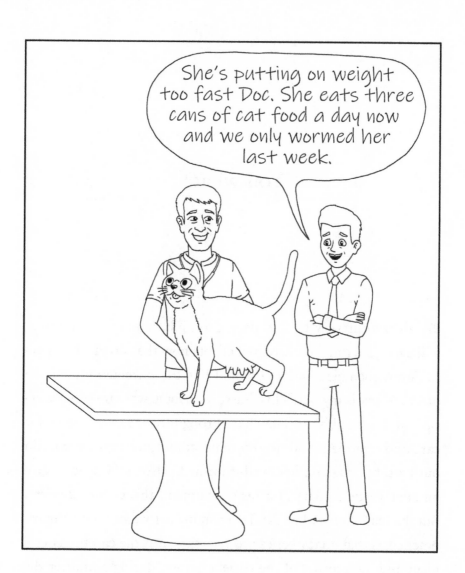

You what?

We all try our very best to do a good job, hoping that nothing will ever go wrong. I always tell clients now that I treat their pets as family members and as I would like to be treated myself. To me, their pet is my pet. This reassures people who are often worried, and justifiably so. They have brought their sick pet to us for care and treatment and need to have confidence that we will do our best, be proactive and well-informed. Also, if we need to give an anaesthetic as part of a pet's treatment, this creates anxiety. But the reality nowadays, and even in my early days of veterinary practice, is that anaesthetics are very safe. It is the careful assessment and monitoring of the patient before, during and after the anaesthetic that is the critical thing. If the patient is high risk, they need to be assessed carefully and the client advised of the risks. It is rare now that we run into any major complications. However, a high-risk patient needs extra care and monitoring. The client must be fully informed and on board.

The same care needs to be taken with a surgical procedure. Does the patient really need it? What are the risks and benefits of the procedure? Most surgical outcomes in experienced hands are excellent, provided there is careful planning, good surgical technique and aftercare.

In saying that, even with the best of intentions and care, things can still occasionally not go as planned. When that happens, it is the steps we take to correct an error, or prevent it from worsening, that are important.

Mistakes do happen. Twice over forty years I have seen the wrong leg operated on. The first time involved a small dog that needed its ACL (anterior cruciate ligament) repaired. When the client arrived to collect the patient and the dog was carried out to them in the waiting room, the client suddenly realised the error and, obviously shocked, let fly with 'You've operated on the wrong leg!' There was a tremendous outburst of yelling in a waiting room full of people.

Now, unfortunately, but fortunately in this case, the dog needed both ACL ligaments operated on as they were both badly ruptured. It was just a matter of staging the surgeries and doing one first, waiting a few months, then operating on the second leg. So, in the end, it did not matter so much. But the legs were operated on in the reverse order.

The second case involved a bone biopsy. The dog had some X-ray abnormality in a leg bone and needed a bone biopsy or sample taken for diagnosis. In this case the wrong leg was biopsied. The veterinarian was devastated, extremely embarrassed and apologetic. The clients were extremely understanding and very nice about it, which was fortunate, so there was no problem. In fact, the clients only ever wanted to see that veterinarian when they visited the clinic in future! Perhaps they thought he'd be extra careful.

It's in the bag

I had just arrived at work one morning when I got a call to a farm north-west of Napier in the region of Patoka, about forty minutes' drive from Napier. It was a nice sunny spring day, although slightly cool with a gentle breeze. These were the days when it was good to escape from the clinic and the intensity of companion-animal practice. You could drive with the car windows down and breathe in the fresh spring air and take joy from the newborn lambs and calves running about in the paddocks or keeping close to mum. This was the weather that farmers wanted at this time of year for all sorts of reasons.

It was school holidays and often farm calls in spring had the added interest of the kids tagging along on the tractor or farm quad bike with the parents, usually Dad. The younger the age, the more wide-eyed they often were at the proceedings.

Vic had phoned my receptionist Anne and said he needed a hand to calve a cow. Jasmine had been straining for twenty minutes but not produced anything. Vic had attempted to assist Jasmine without success, and fortunately the calf was still alive.

'OK, I'll be there in forty-five minutes,' I said, and I was on my way.

When I arrived, Jasmine was very bright and patiently waiting in the pen.

There was Vic, his wife Elisa, and their two children, Jack and his younger sister Sophie.

'What a stunning day it is,' I said, suddenly realising it probably wasn't so good for them having to call me out for a calving problem. But they all politely agreed.

What a great job it would be if every call-out were on a day such as this. Sadly, that was not the case, so best to enjoy it while I could.

The wide-eyed curiosity of the young ones was intense today and as I kitted up with the calving gown, gloves and lube, Vic and Elisa were giving Jack and Sophie a run-down of what I was doing.

I examined Jasmine and thankfully there was plenty of room for the calf to pass through her pelvis. And yes, the calf was alive. There were not very strong contractions coming from Jasmine and I thought that she would benefit from an injection of oxytocin and calcium and an infusion of electrolytes. So, we set up an intravenous drip to run the electrolytes and calcium in and gave the oxytocin intramuscularly, to assist with the uterine contractions.

It was not very long at all before Jasmine produced some very good contractions and shortly after that she gave birth to a fine healthy female calf enclosed in the amniotic sac as usual. We moved in and broke the birth sac or the bag of waters surrounding the calf so she could breathe and left the rest to Jasmine.

With that Jack piped up. 'Daddy, why is the calf born in a plastic bag?'

Afterthoughts

As with people in many careers, a veterinarian gets on with doing the job. In clinical practice that involves dealing with emergencies and illnesses, both acute and chronic. As in human health care and the other caring professions in general, more of our work now involves preventative medicine and client education. Emergency work is still a large part of clinical practice, and always will be. There is something very satisfying in helping our furry friends to better health while at the same time witnessing the relief and gratitude of the pet owner. It gives us immense pleasure and reinforces our personal sense of purpose.

We are commonly asked how we manage to do our jobs. Many people wonder how we cope emotionally and psychologically with the rigours of the job and particularly the euthanasia of pets. Clients will often say, 'I don't know how you do your job; it must be very hard.' This is especially true when you have had a long association with the pet and client, or when we are faced with a family or pet owner who is extremely upset. However, whether you are dealing with an accident or emergency, or the euthanasia of a beloved pet, it is all part of the job that we accept when we graduate. If we have done our very best, and approached the situation with sympathy and empathy, then that is all we can do. Moreover, it is a privilege and honour to be able to assist at this difficult time and to alleviate any further suffering. Rather than prolonging suffering that can only end in death, we are able to avoid suffering and hasten a painless death. Of course, everyone has their own opinion and set of values regarding the end of life, and that is to be respected. However, with our animal patients who cannot speak for themselves and have no control over this, it is up to us to advise and assist in the most humane manner possible. It is often the animal's owner who knows when the time is right to make the difficult end-of-life decision, and we are there to support them at this very difficult time.

On a lighter note, veterinarians also manage to get their share of laughs, despite our professional responsibilities, which we take very seriously.

Still, as you can see from some of these stories, there are many light-hearted moments. It is often in hindsight that we can fully appreciate the moment, or see the humour in a situation. At the time there is often a job to be done and an outcome to achieve, and the humour may not be appropriate nor able to be appreciated or enjoyed. There are situations where the veterinarian and the client can both have a good laugh together, especially on farm calls, even if the humour is at someone's expense – often that of the veterinarian. Our well-qualified and very dedicated veterinary nurses, who are the backbone of our profession, keep us on our toes, and a few laughs with them can lighten our day immensely.

One of the regrets that I personally have is not stopping often enough throughout my career and taking a moment to reflect on the good outcomes that are achieved in just doing my job, and on a job well done. For me personally, this would have helped reinforce the sense of purpose and self-worth that is critical to wellbeing, inner satisfaction, and calm. I think we all need to pat ourselves on the back more often when a job is well done. Take the time to appreciate what you have to offer and have offered. If you do this, it can also be good for those who work with you and support you – your colleagues and workmates.

Most of all we shouldn't forget our furry friends. How fortunate we all are to have them in our lives. And what job can you think of where you go to work every day to be met, by and large, by a barrage of happy, unconditionally loving faces? Most of our routine patients – but of course not all – are happy to visit us. In the case of our canine friends, you could argue that this is in part related to the ready supply of treats behind the counter, but nevertheless a glass-half-full disposition is the rule rather than the exception, treat or no treat.

About the author

Mike Small was born and grew up in New Zealand. Mike qualified and graduated as a veterinarian from Massey University, Palmerston North, New Zealand in the 1980s. After working in New Plymouth for six months, he owned a mixed-animal veterinary practice in Napier for nine years, before moving to Auckland where he spent most of his working life as a partner in a companion-animal practice. His special veterinary interests include surgery and ultrasound. He has been involved in and acted as a trustee of a dog rescue trust for many years. Outside of work, his family is a big part of his life and he is an avid runner, cyclist, hiker, traveller, and amateur chef. He is currently living in Melbourne, Australia, with his partner and their miniature schnauzer dog Elisa and Burmese cat Luca.

CPSIA information can be obtained
at www.ICGtesting.com
Printed in the USA
LVHW030241130121
676282LV00004B/255